Live Pain FREE!

Proven Methods You Can Use
To Start Feeling Better Today

Proven Methods You Can Use To Start Feeling Better Today

Live Pain FREE!

Dr. Mark Wiley

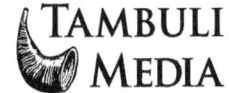
TAMBULI MEDIA

www.TambuliMedia.com
Spring House, PA USA

DISCLAIMER

The information contained in this book is meant to educate the reader, and is in no way intended to provide medical, financial, legal or any other services for individual problems or circumstances. We encourage readers to seek advice from competent professionals for personal health, financial and legal needs.

First Published August 10, 2016 by Tambuli Media
Copyright 2016 by Mark V. Wiley
ISBN-10: 1-943155-20-8
ISBN-13: 978-1-943155-20-0
Library of Congress Control Number: 2016949128

All Rights Reserved. No part of this publication may be reproduced or utilized in any form or by any means, electronic or mechanical, including photocopying, recording, or by any information storage and retrieval system, without prior written permission from the Publisher or Author.

Cover & Interior by Summer Bonne

FOREWORD

BY MICHAEL MALISZEWSKI, PHD

I am pleased to write a foreword to Dr. Mark Wiley's new book, *Live Pain Free!*, as I have known Mark for over 20 years. We have shared parallel paths of investigation, seeking out the most effective techniques, procedures, programs, and practitioners professing to have the best and most comprehensive approach to pain management and control, leading to reduction in severity of pain conditions and symptoms. I believe Mark's approach to pain management is "cutting edge," offering the most progressive focus available today as compared to other strategies currently present in the healthcare field.

A quick note regarding my background to add credence to my statements and position. I received my training as a clinical psychologist at the University of Chicago. After a traditional background, I went on to develop the world's largest single-site behavioral medicine program at the Diamond Headache

Clinic in Chicago, a setting which treated some 20,000 patients annually for headache pain and related disorders using an approach known as Accelerated Behavioral Medicine (ABM). Compared to other pain treatment programs available that involved anywhere from two weeks to several months of training to participate, the design of the ABM program was to assess pain conditions and offer the most rapid way to reduce pain through nonpharmacological, psychological strategies, with a maximum time being three hours. After some eight years of developing the ABM program, I then became associated with the psychology/psychiatry department at Massachusetts General Hospital (MGH)/Harvard Medical School, serving as a consultant at that setting for 20 years. I am currently a member of the Integrative Medicine Task Force at Spaulding Hospital in Boston, another Harvard-based hospital affiliated with MGH, in addition to private practice consultation. In addition, I received grants to travel and conduct field research on indigenous healing traditions throughout nearly a dozen Asian countries, in addition to investigating pain programs throughout the USA and Europe.

Sharing a similar thirst for knowledge and discovery, Mark Wiley and I became familiar with one another's work, research, and writings, recognizing how truly limited the background was to other programs and practitioners offering pain relief solutions to their clients. Our parallel approaches entailed what might be termed an "evidence based practice" to testing the most viable and successful strategies to pain control within ourselves and with our clients.

I cannot emphasize enough the importance of the approach Dr. Wiley presents to you in this book. This is not simply a compendium of techniques currently popular in the literature or found in online searches. Nor is it an advertisement to argue the superiority of one method, approach, or program over another. It goes much deeper. A basic tenet is that a combination of various therapies and approaches offer the best chance for improvement. But even more relevant, it stresses the importance of self-administration of pain-relieving techniques where the pain sufferer takes control of his or her conditions(s) directly and initiates and pursues an individualized, self-design module rather than relying exclusively on some external program or practitioner to alleviate the pain for them. A psychologist might describe it as a shift in locus of control from external agent and back to the persons themselves. This is unique among the most popular program today which offer highly publicized approaches and outcomes in the media but which are also quite expensive in terms of costs (financial as well as time invested).

Live Pain Free! is a welcome breath of fresh air for acute and chronic pain sufferers everywhere who either need a little help or are at their wit's end. All it takes is the motivated individual who wants to lead a healthy and pain-free lifestyle with minimal inconveniences and a positive opportunity for further growth and freedom from pain.

CONTENTS

Introduction: My Personal Pain Experience and How I Can Help You 1

Chapter 1: When the Pain Comes... What Do I Do?.......... 7

Chapter 2: What Type of Pain Do I Have? 15
    The Secret Key to Easy Pain Relief............................ 15

Chapter 3: The Pain-Sleep Connection and the Hidden Sleep Wrecker.. 23

Chapter 4: The Fibromyalgia Puzzle – Pain Relief Starting Today 31
    Exercise to Boost Energy and Brain Health – and Banish Fibromyalgia Pain 36
    Fibromyalgia Relief in Daily Qigong Practice 40
    Beyond Fibro: Soothe Nerve Pain Naturally 43
    EXTRA: Zap Your Pain Away with FSM Therapy 47

Chapter 5: What to Do About Your Pain in the Neck 55
    EXTRA: Scraping Pain Away................................ 64

Chapter 6: Six Natural Ways to Reduce Acute Pain and Muscle Spasms 69

Chapter 7: Natural Painkilling Solutions 77
    Three Super Spices that Knock Out Pain 82
    Try DMSO and Wipe Out Pain and Inflammation 86
    Magnificent Magnesium 90
    EXTRA: Use Chinese Topical Treatments for Pain Relief 93
    Do You Have Peppermint Oil in Your Medicine Cabinet? 99

Chapter 8: Dealing With Low Back Pain, the World's No. 1 Health Problem 105
    How to Stop Back Pain and Save Your Spine from Swayback 110
    Power Through Work or Play with NO Back Pain.... 115

Chapter 9: Joint Pain Gone! Easy Tricks to Relieve Knee, Carpal Tunnel, Hand and Wrist Pain 121
    Natural Approaches for Alleviating Knee Pain 121
    "Help, I Can't Type!" or How to Get Carpal Tunnel Relief Starting Today 128
    Easy Relief for the Heel Pain of Plantar Fasciitis 131
    Vanquish Joint Pain on the Cellular Level 136

Chapter 10: Real Solutions to the Migraine Puzzle 141
    Migraine Pain: Stopping this Gateway to a Stroke 149
    The Best Nutrients and Vitamins for Migraine
    Relief 158
    Controlling Headache Triggers 163
    EXTRA: Spray Away Migraine Pain? 167

Chapter 11: Reversing Arthritis 171
    Top 10 Arthritis Mistakes 171

Chapter 12: Chinese Medicine for Physical Injuries 179

Chapter 13: When Natural Therapy Isn't Enough 187

Chapter 14: When Pain Won't Go Away, it May be Tension Myositis Syndrome 195

Chapter 15: The Newest – and Oldest – in Alternative Anti-Pain Therapies 201
    Acupuncture Offers Better Pain Relief 201
    Step Into the Doorway to Pain Relief 206
    Align Body, Mind and Gravity to Banish Pain 214
    Awareness and Pain Relief Through "Opposite"
    Movement 218
    Banish Pain and Stiffness with the Muscle Energy
    Technique 223

Afterword: Take Control of Your Pain 233

About the Author 239

Index 243

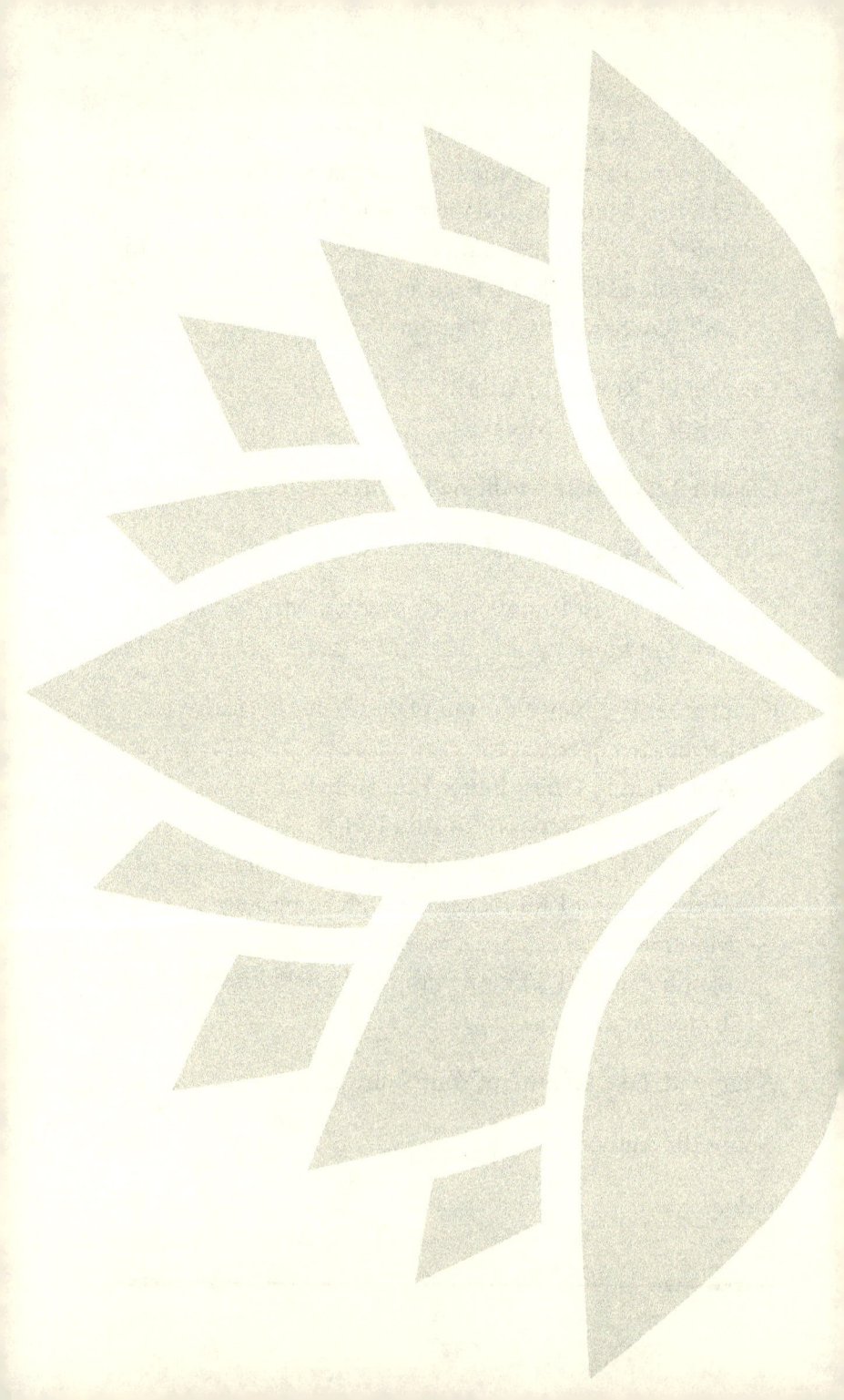

INTRODUCTION

MY PERSONAL PAIN EXPERIENCE AND HOW I CAN HELP YOU

I got into natural healing practices because I suffered decades of chronic pain. This encompassed daily headaches and migraines, musculoskeletal pain, hip pain, muscle spasms, trigger points and arthritis. I found that medicine could help me with short-term reduction of inflammation and pain, but was not helpful in the long run. Actually, in my experience, by taking so many pain meds, I helped cover up the pain so well I did not feel compelled to address the pain in other, more beneficial, ways.

In addition to seeing dozens of medical doctors and specialists, I also consulted with a stable of expert practitioners in various fields of mind/body and alternative medicine. I experienced acupuncture for opening the blocked energy channels, herbs for increasing energy and reducing inflammation, diet for lowering inflammation and a dozen bodywork systems for relieving muscle pain and correcting skeletal misalignment. In addition, I tried bio-feedback and electro-stimulation. Even psychic surgery. You name it and I did it.

But none of these methods (modern or traditional, scientific or natural) helped me in the long run.

Over the years, through first hand experience and study, I can to understand that the reasons for this long-term ineffectiveness are rooted in several factors.

THE MEDICATION PROBLEM

Taking medication, both prescription or over-the-counter, is good for short-term care. If you're getting a cold or can't sleep, or have a sprained ankle, pills can help reduce the symptoms linked to those ailments. But that medication is not a long-term solution and does not provide corrective support – only symptomatic relief.

THE PRACTITIONER PROBLEM

Going to see a practitioner of any health modality (be it acupuncture, chiropractic, physical therapy, etc.) can be a good solution for acute pain. Practitioners can "get in there" and help adjust things in a way we, on our own or by taking medicine, cannot. A chiropractor can align the spine, and an acupuncturist can open energy blockages. A physical therapist can help strengthen weak processes. However, by their very nature, all hands-on healing modalities place us in a secondary (receiving) position and are therefore, on their own, not good long-term solutions to pain relief. Our own health and wellness and cannot be dependent on another person.

THE DIETARY PROBLEM

Diet is a main component in health and in disease. Eating well-balanced, organic foods is essential to good health and vibrant well-being. When you're in pain, anti-inflammatory foods and pain-relieving foods and spices can help you get through the acute injury. However, dietary changes, by themselves, are not strong enough to ease severe pain. Moreover, diet does not do enough to correct pain caused by muscle or vertebral imbalances, blunt force trauma or trigger points. However, diet IS a vital part of the pain-relief equation.

CONSEQUENTLY...

My own experience demonstrates that, depending on the severity of the acute injury and length of the chronic condition, a combination of all these therapies produces the best improvement.

Taking analgesics or anti-inflammatory drugs can really help you get past the severe pain of serious injury. To avoid liver and kidney damage, you should switch to less potent drugs and, over time, it's advisable to switch fully to herbs and supplements. Along the way, changing your diet to avoid inflammation-promoting foods (sugar, wheat, nightshades) and consume more anti-inflammatory foods (aromatic spices, ginger and turmeric) can help. Seeing a hands-on practitioner also helps the body start correcting itself, loosening muscles, improving range of motion, opening energy channels, aligning the spine and more. But over time you need to learn various stretching and trigger-point release methods that you can do on your own so that you are in control of your wellbeing. You can then self-administer pain-relieving techniques at the start of an issue instead of waiting, depending on others, and allowing it to become chronic.

This kind of comprehensive approach is great and more powerful than any single approach. However, it's not always enough to be fully satisfying. When I suffered, I constantly wanted it to be over. I did not want to have to wait every other day or bi-weekly for a massage or chiropractic adjustment. I didn't want to keep taking pills. Just wanting faster results for most of my problems did not produce quicker relief. As a result, my pain transformed from acute to chronic. My body learned a new pattern – and I seemed stuck with it.

That's why I've spent most of my focus, since I was about 13 to becoming a healer… the last 34 years studying, experimenting, discovering, learning and practicing how to heal pain – first for my myself and then for others. At the time of this writing I am 47 and still searching for the best the world has to offer for natural pain relief. I travel constantly in search of new information and old practices that I've missed. I read medical studies every day looking for interesting clinical trials and keeping current on trends.

In this book I want to show you everything I've learned thus far, so you can use it as a guide to relieve and get past any type of pain you're experiencing so you can live your life again, the way you want to. Living pain free is your birthright. Start reclaiming it today. I'll show you how.

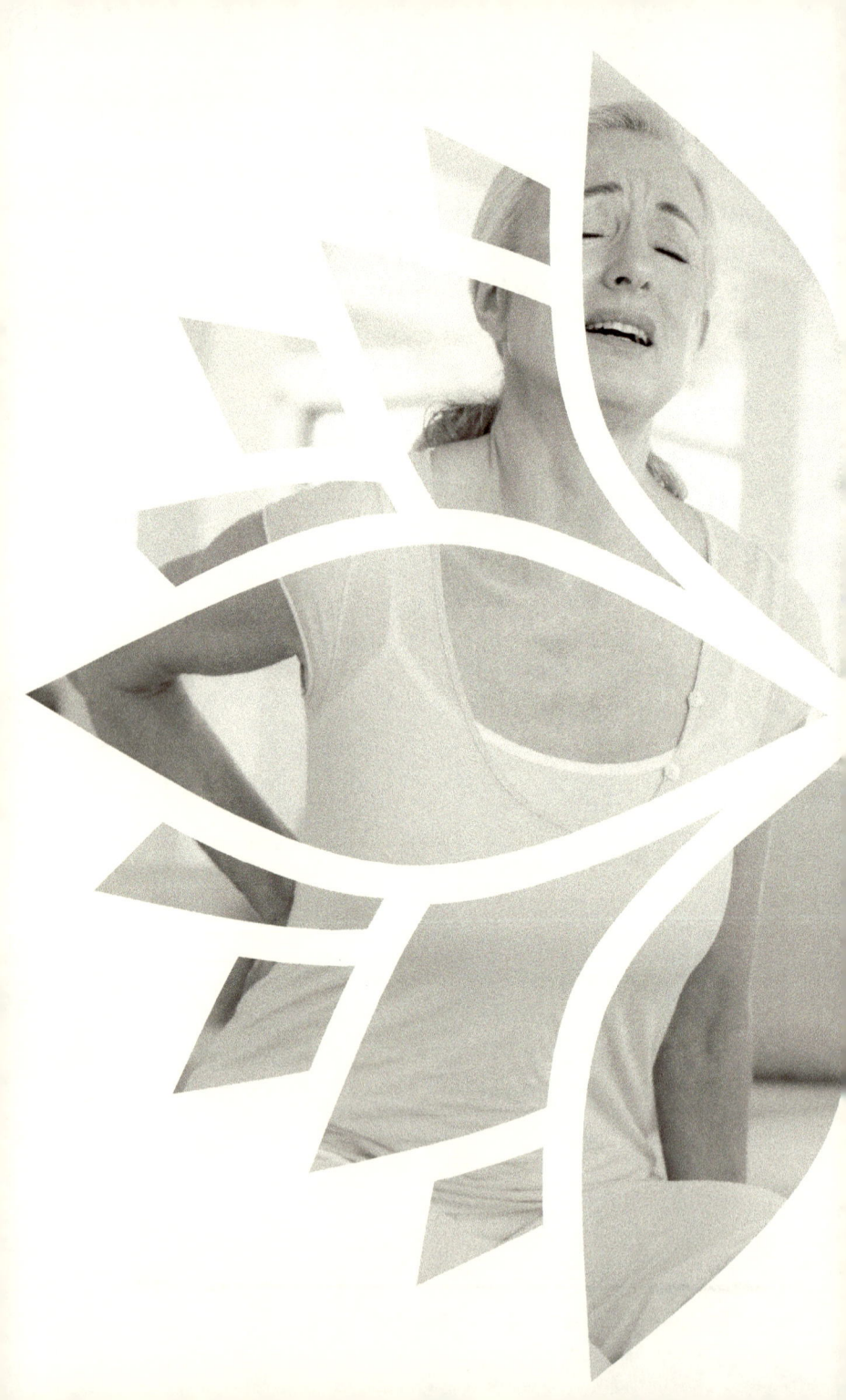

CHAPTER 1

WHEN THE PAIN COMES... WHAT DO I DO?

From early on, you are taught to "manage," "mask the symptoms of" and "live with" your poor health conditions.

This is perverse.

It goes against our homeostatic (self-balancing) nature. What's more, despite lackluster results, too many people keep following the practices of a healthcare system that simply has not delivered on its promises.

Are we doing this because we don't realize it's not working? Surely, our daily chronic pain and suffering is the indication it's not working.

Simply put, mainstream medicine fails to eradicate our everyday pains, illnesses and diseases. It fails because it is passive and reactionary and thus unable to prevent you from experiencing chronic health conditions like heart disease, diabetes, hyper-tension, obesity, stress, anxiety, depression, headache, back pain, tendonitis and hundreds of others.

And this model will always fall short because it uses disease as its basis of finding health.

That is, you go and see your primary care physician when you are ill, the doctor diagnoses your illness, labels the disease, then prescribes a protocol for treating that disease or the symptoms you are suffering.

Your personal health issues are "managed" by prescription medication, various therapies and surgery.

Natural treatment can also fall into this category, if the approach is relief of symptoms and not correction of underlying (root) causes.

While treating symptoms of pain and inflammation are necessary for immediate relief, it must be done as an intermediary step while implementing a truly corrective approach.

After all, any model based simply on symptomatic relief (whether modern or traditional) can never hope to resolve your daily pain problems.

Your best course of action is to carefully analyze the source of your pain and use natural pain relief methods to stem the discomfort.

Pain can originate from many sources: You're on the run and seized by a spasm in your neck. The stress of the day triggers a migraine. Or you overexert yourself, and now your back is out.

You are a busy person and can't let these ailments derail your day or your week, even if they are intensely painful. So you head to the nearest drugstore and look for quick relief in a bottle, a patch or a cream.

When you get there, you are overwhelmed with choices. You look at packaging; recall past experiences and mull over product advertising claims before reaching for the most popular brand and hoping for the best.

Several hours later, you're still in pain and you take another dose of the over-the-counter (OTC) remedy. Later, you experience stomach discomfort and gastrointestinal irritation from those pills. And your body still hurts.

COMPLICATED ANSWERS

If you're like millions of other Americans, you have at least one (and probably several) chronic health concerns. For many, it's a pain-related ailment. Back pain is reported as the number one reason people visit their primary care physician. Headaches and joint pain rank up there, too. I am often asked which OTC remedy is best for pain. The answer, however, is not a simple one.

Like many of you, I am both amazed and dumbfounded by the volume of pain products on the market. A short walk down any store's supplement aisle is soon overwhelming if one is hoping to find relief for symptoms. How is it that there can be so many products for pain? Some block the pain receptors, while others reduce inflammation. Also offered: Topical pain patches, heat therapy, cold therapy and on and on.

Which treatment is the right one to use for your pain or discomfort?

The biggest issue to understand is that no individual product is suitable for every pain problem, despite marketing and accepted wisdom. For example, if you have neck pain, should you choose ibuprofen (an anti-inflammatory) or naproxen (an analgesic)? Many people think they are identical. After all, they both relieve pain. Yet, most people find that one product works better for them than the other. (This fact alone is a clear hint that not all products work as well for the same general issue.)

So while Motrin® and Aleve® both help reduce pain sensations for a period of time, they do so from different mechanisms.

If your pain is the result of inflammation, then Motrin® matched with a cool-therapy patch, cream or compress is a relatively better choice. However, if your pain results from trigger points, Aleve®, coupled with a heat-therapy cream, patch or pad is a relatively better option. I say relatively because neither OTC pain reliever is natural, and either can harm the body when used for an extended period of time.

DIFFERENT CAUSES

When pain symptoms are felt in the neck, the cause of the pain is not the same as it is for back pain. As a basic rule, however, inflammation should be reduced while spasms and trigger points should be released. Applying heat to pain originating from inflammation makes the symptoms worse and applying cold to already constricted muscles makes those symptoms worse. Spending a moment to discern the pain syndrome (collection of symptoms) before making your pain-relieving selection goes a long way towards quickening the results you desire – without aggravating symptoms or making the ailment more painful.

The idea here is that one size does not fit all, thus no one pain product is best for all types of pain. Don't mindlessly grab a product off the shelf when you're experiencing symptoms just because that product worked for a friend, you saw a convincing ad or it's on sale. Think the situation through first – and then decide which (if any) product is a good choice.

Is your pain throbbing… the site of the pain red and swollen? Do you have restricted range of motion? These questions are relevant to understanding the source of the pain, which itself is a symptom of a larger imbalance. Until the cause of the pain is addressed, the pain will inevitably return and you'll need more meds to ease the discomfort.

Another problem with OTC pain relief is that these products are only effective for the limited time the remedy is active in your body. This is usually between two and four hours. After that, their effects wear off and you need to take more. The serious problem here is that if the product is not the most appropriate to your pain syndrome, you can actually be damaging your body while not even truly helping the issue. More importantly, if the product works on symptomatic relief (which most do) and not on changing the problem itself (which most don't), then you risk becoming chronically dependent on the product. This can lead to serious problems for your stomach lining, digestive tract, liver and kidneys. All the while your original pain problem continues.

REALITIES

While I advocate natural health products, I am realistic in my expectations of them. Most natural products for pain are best used as preventive measures or at the very first sign of pain symptoms. Natural pain products like arnica, turmeric, capsicum, angelica root, feverfew, camphor and others are safe and gentle on the system. However, they generally are not strong enough to be much help during severe pain that is in full swing. Also, like OTC pain meds, these are each specific for different kinds of pain-related symptoms. Arnica is appropriate for topical inflammation and turmeric for systemic inflammation; capsicum for muscle spasm and angelica root to quicken blood stagnation and so on. Again, even with natural products, it is advised to first examine your pain type, then consider the related symptoms that are also occurring and look for a solution to address the overall pain syndrome you are experiencing in that moment.

ENVIRONMENTAL ROOTS

For your body to experience pain of any kind, there must be an environment within it that allows the symptoms to take hold and cause you discomfort. This means that if your muscles are supple and blood is moving through them in the appropriate way, you should not experience muscle tightness, strain or trigger points. However, because of poor diet, lack of stretching and exercise and sitting for long periods of time, the resting length of muscles shortens and less blood moves through them more slowly, allowing toxins to build in the tissue. Those events cause pain and trigger points to manifest.

Instead of unconsciously reaching for an anti-inflammatory pain reliever (for example), you should be doing several things that can solve your problem:

- Correcting the habit that creates the problem.
- Changing the environment in the muscle housing the problem.
- Using the appropriate pain-relieving product.
- Preventing a cycle of looking to short-term relief from the wrong product that will likely become chronic.

To remedy pain, you must think about your pain and try to discern what kind it is.

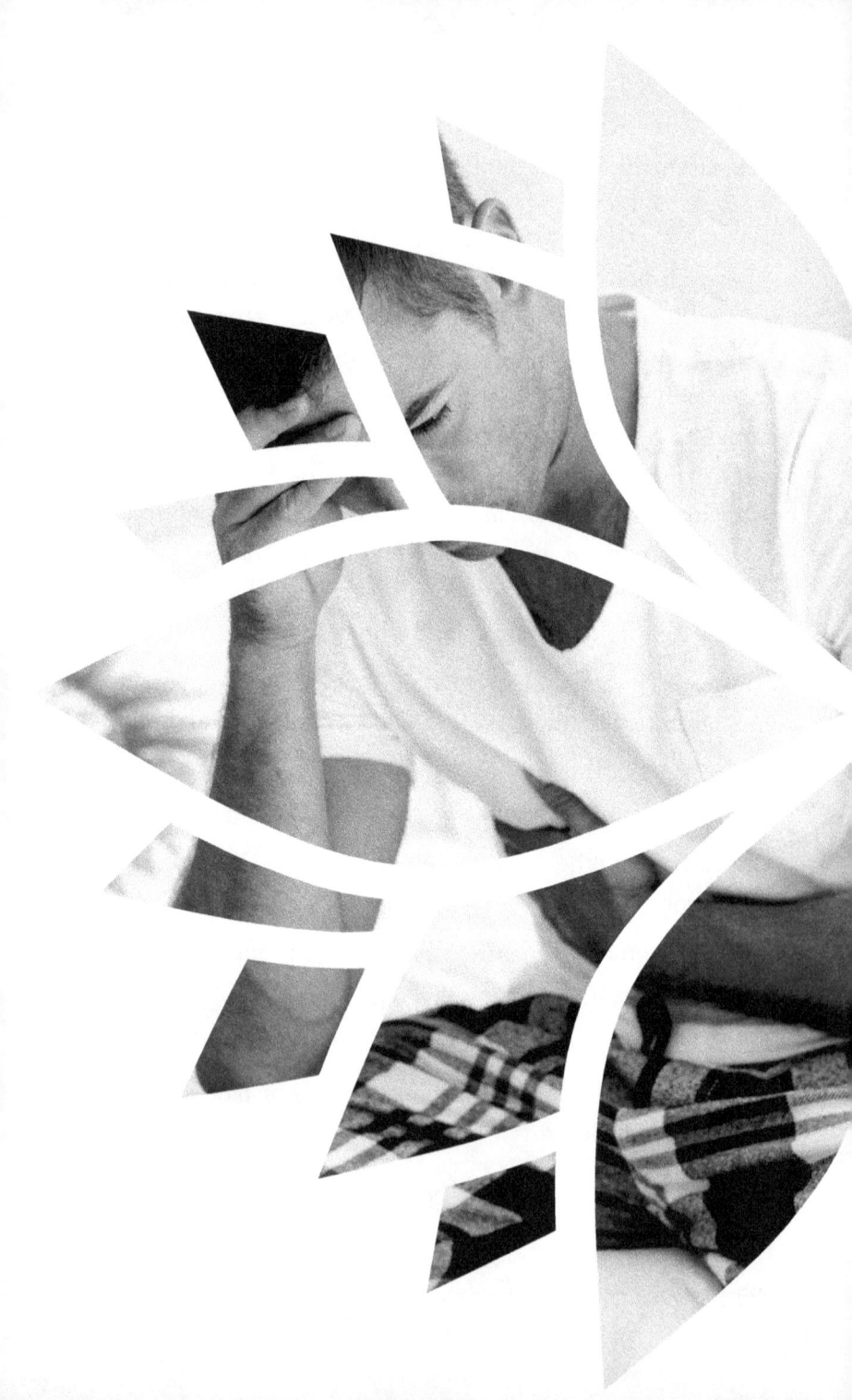

CHAPTER 2

WHAT TYPE OF PAIN DO I HAVE?

*P*ain is no joking matter… but neither is it something to describe vaguely.

If I had to name the first reason that some people experience faster pain relief than others, I would say it's because of "specifics." By this I mean how specifically one is able to describe their pain or condition to a practitioner – or to themselves.

Challenges for healthcare practitioners and take-charge pain relief seekers arise when non-specific words are used to describe symptoms of their condition. Specifics are always what are needed to lead one in the right direction for relief or cure. This is derived in part from an extensive physical examination and patient consultation.

Part of this health history and health assessment is based on types of sensations felt in the body, either as constant pain, throbbing or distension, etc. And each of these holds different meaning in our understanding of the problem and formation of a diagnosis.

Thus, general adjectives like "painful" and "hurting" just don't give enough insight into what you may actually be suffering from. And the type of pain points the way to the type of treatment best used to alleviate it.

For faster results, you must come to know your pain by "examining" it. Take some time to "feel" it or "listen" to it, or "fully experience" it without a distracted mind. Of course, there are many types and causes of pain and stiffness. To give you a hand, let me describe seven of the most common. I sincerely hope this list will help you become better acquainted with your own pain… and thus be better equipped to find a reliable therapy. Some of the terms used to describe are from traditional Chinese medicine (TCM) and may seem "strange." No worries; by the end of the book you will be very familiar with them.

Inflammation: This generally occurs around the joints and involves stasis (a slowing or stoppage) of fluids (water retention) or reaction to stimuli (sprain or strain). Inflammation can be caused by heat syndromes, blood count changes and fluid deficiencies.

Swelling: This generally occurs around the ankles or wrists, but can also occur on the face or any part of the body. Its symptom is stasis, or collection of fluids leading to puffiness. The area may be either hot and reddish or cold and whitish – depending on whether the swelling is due to heat or cold.

Numbness and Tingling: These are caused by nerve entrapment or dysfunction or by a lack of circulation in the body. It will occur when blood flow is deficient either from an external obstruction, or from some anemic or biological blood deficiency. External causes can be from compressed nerves in the spine, from holding a limb in a fixed position too long or from sleeping on or resting against a limb for an extended period of time.

Heaviness and Stiffness: These are characterized by a dull and nagging sensation in the body. It's an achy feeling that is made worse by cold and damp weather and when circulation is slow, such as in the morning hours. It mostly affects the joints, neck and back, and is often temporarily relieved by hot showers or baths, where blood is able to circulate better.

Distending and Throbbing Pain: These types of pain are like something is pushing from the inside out. It's a pressing and exploding pain that tends to beat in tandem with the pulse. It is mostly caused by qi or energy stagnation, wherein energy is moving but going nowhere – except up and down in one location. Thus, you get a fixed pain that throbs and causes distension of an area.

Stabbing Pain: This type of pain is caused either by blood stasis or both qi (energy) and blood stasis (sluggishness). Since blood promotes energy and energy is the motive force behind blood, stabbing pain generally includes problems with both. Think about a muscle spasm in the neck or shoulders that feel worse with pressure.

Dull, Lingering Pain: This type of pain is not so severe, yet it doesn't seem to go away. Migraine sufferers and sciatica sufferers generally describe a dull pain that lingers after their acute symptoms have subsided. Dull pains tend to become worse with exhaustion and when hunger is present, as the body is weakening and the pain tolerance system is low. Dull pain is caused by a general deficiency of energy and/or blood, such as follows a lingering illness or injury.

What is the best remedy? How do you overcome or change the environment that allows pain to persist, and what behavior is responsible for that environment? Change the behavior and you can change the environment within your body and consequently limit the occurrence of pain and reduce it from chronic to acute (or remove it altogether).

Natural products and methods are always best, but in times of acute flare-up or chronic conditions, a little help from other sources can get you to the point where the natural products can do their work most effectively. However, if you grab the wrong OTC product, your problem may worsen.

THE SECRET KEY TO EASY PAIN RELIEF

Pain usually comes and goes. But when it comes and stays, you often end up with chronic pain – the bane of conventional medicine, which is good at emergency and acute medical care but highly unsuccessful in dealing with chronic pain.

There are many therapies available for pain reduction. But in the end, many people end up with a "pain management" regimen. This should not be the case.

So before I show you anything else, I want to reveal to you one method you can try that might just relieve almost all your pain.

THE PROBLEM WITH FASCIA

What I didn't know as a kid, teen or even as a young man was that the human body is wrapped in connective tissue called fascia. Found 2 mm under the skin, this connective tissue encases your entire body, every organ and cell, like a massive spider web. Fascia connects every part of you, holds every part in place and gives you your shape.

But the problem with fascia is that it sticks.

When you are fit, or at least not injured, fascia slides, expands and contracts with your body. As you twist and turn, the fascia, encasing various parts of your body, moves over, under or along with your entire body. The body works well, you feel good, range of motion is correct and there is no pain.

However, either through injury (torn muscle, sprained ankle) or repetitive inactivity (sitting too long, working at a desk), the joints and body parts not in full use become immobilized. Fascia gets sticky and adheres when range of motion is not used (think of frozen shoulder that results from having your arm in a sling).

Essentially, fascia can stick to itself, gluing in place muscles and joints that should be free to move in their normal ranges. When their movement is restricted, pain results that limits physicality and quality of life. Then, pain from injury or inactivity changes from being acute to chronic. Fascia holds the injury in place and prolongs it.

WHAT YOU CAN DO

The solution to this pain problem is to take ownership of your injury and your recovery. It's easy and it's free. In addition to any medications, ice/heat therapies, hands-on therapies or practitioner practices you are using to recover, you need to keep your fascia at the injury site from sticking. This means doing things every day to ensure it stays free and to break up what is or has stuck. You should do this even though you're seeing a practitioner or taking pain relieving medication, too.

Here is how to do it:

- **Keep moving, if only slowly.** Walking, bending and squatting are all ways you can move and articulate the major joints in the body. Maintaining movement keeps blood flowing, fluids in motion and joints moving.

- **Rotate the joints.** You cannot get frozen shoulders when you continually move your shoulder joints. Loosen up all your joints by rotating them forward then backward for a count of 20, several times per day. Start from the head and work down to the toes.

- **Stretch the muscles.** This helps keep the body loose and limber, moves in fresh blood and oxygen to problem areas and expels toxins from tissues. When injuries occur, muscles generally tighten around the area as a natural means of protection. It's not healthy to remain so protected for long periods, so stretching slowly and gently each day will help the body realize when it is OK to "let go."

- **Roll your body on a foam roller.** Massage is great but can be expensive and requires the services of a massage therapist. You can get similar results on your own by using a foam roller. These are dense lengths of foam that you lie on and roll on, pressing against all parts of your body and limbs. The pressure of your bodyweight against the foam roller compresses muscles, massages tissues, releases toxins and allows the movement of body fluids essential for repair. Because rolling is gentle, the body does not go into protective mode, as it sometimes does during a deep massage.

- **Get ample sleep every night.** The body repairs and adjusts itself during sleep hours. It's vital to pain relief.

Each of these actions help you reduce pain and help prevent acute pain from becoming chronic. In addition to standard meds and treatments, releasing your fascia is a must.

But speaking of sleep, there's something you should know…

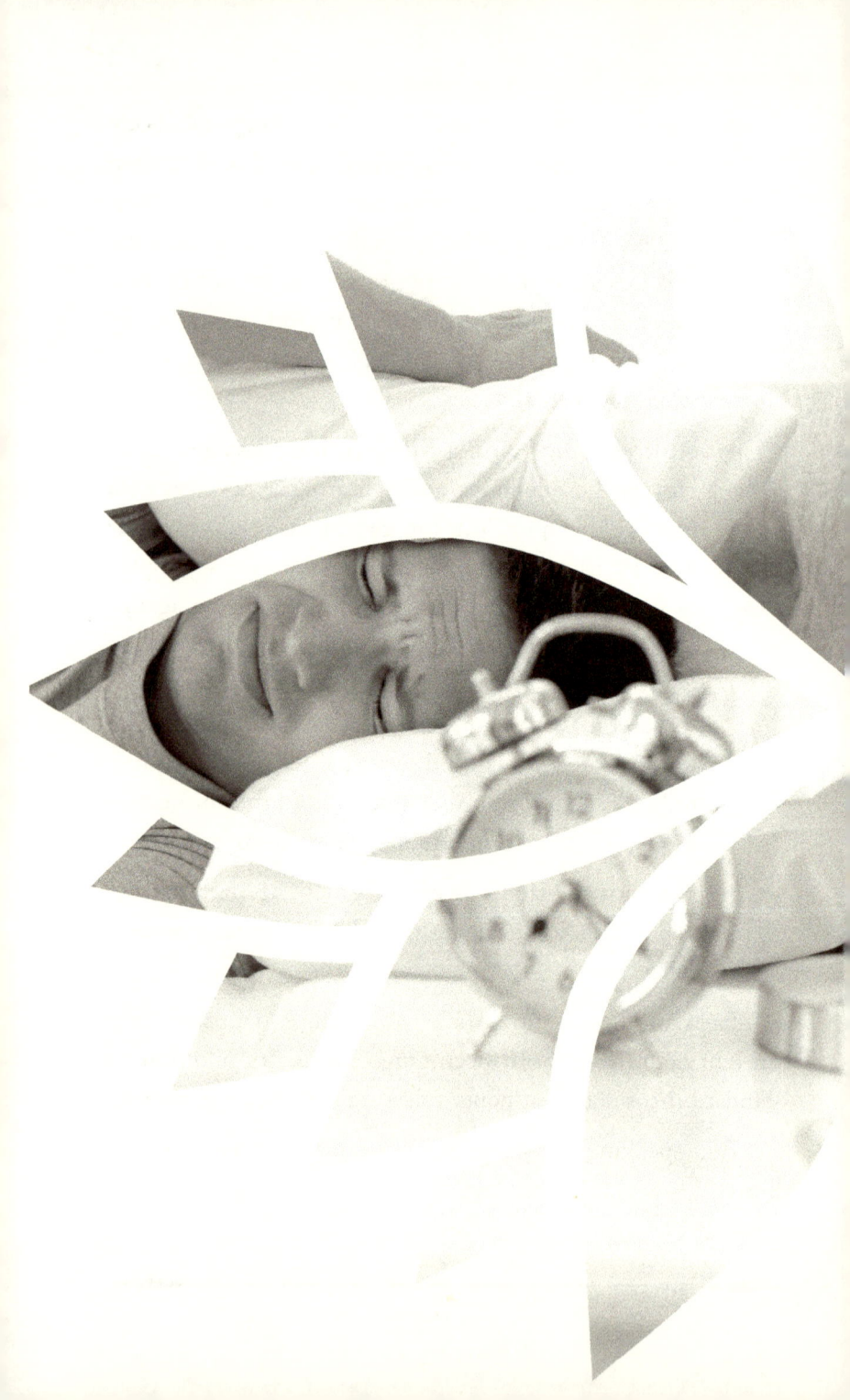

CHAPTER 3

THE PAIN-SLEEP CONNECTION AND THE HIDDEN SLEEP WRECKER

We know that humans need sleep, although it's not clear why. What we do know is that sleep clears toxins from the brain, metabolizes harmful stress hormones, and that it regenerates the body and mind.

Yet, for some reason, the medical establishment does not see the connection between sleep and pain, even though a third of Americans suffer chronic pain, and almost the same number don't get the minimum recommended daily allowance (RDA) of sleep.

Daily sound sleep for eight hours could provide a simple, natural means of pain reduction and prevention. And several studies back this up.

THE PAIN STORY

Pain is a huge problem for the body and the mind and the spirit. There's a real loss of joy for life, reduced physical activity and the onset of depression that often accompany chronic pain and lack of sound sleep.

About 10 years ago the American Pain Foundation conducted a survey that evaluated the impact chronic pain had on over 300 chronic pain sufferers who were taking strong opioids daily to make it through their days.

Here is how the participants responded to the survey:

- 51% felt they had little or no control over their pain.
- 60% said they experience breakthrough pain one or more times daily, severely impacting their quality of life and overall well-being.
- 59% reported an impact on their overall enjoyment of life.
- 77% reported feeling depressed.
- 70% said they have trouble concentrating.
- 74% said their energy level is impacted by their pain.
- 86% reported an inability to sleep well.

Those are not happy responses and certainly no way to live a happy, fulfilled life.

But there is one safe and natural means of reducing pain, and that is getting a solid eight hours of undisturbed sleep per night. Yet, so many of us don't get enough sleep, allowing sleep deprivation to become a co-founder to chronic pain.

THE SLEEP STORY

Sleep deprivation is a serious problem that not only keeps the body from the full recuperation and recovery it needs, but causes accidents, injuries and leads to heart disease and depression.

If people could just get enough sleep, life would be better. The National Institutes of Health (NIH) suggest the following sleep guidelines:

- School-age children = 10 hrs daily.
- Teenagers = 9-10 hrs daily.
- Adults = 7-8 hrs daily.

The problem is, with stress, responsibilities and advances in technology that fragment our attention, sleep hours for all Americans has decreased steadily over the past half-century. In fact, a recent study looked directly at the link between this epidemic of chronic sleep deprivation and the epidemic of chronic pain.

THE PAIN-SLEEP CONNECTION

A recent study published in the online journal PLOS ONE set out to examine the effect sleep had on the physical activity the following day of patients who suffer both chronic pain and insomnia.

For the study, 119 chronic pain patients monitored their sleep and physical activity for a week in their usual sleeping and living environments. The results were very interesting:

"SQ [sleep quality] was the only significant within-person predictor of subsequent physical activity, such that nights of higher sleep quality were followed by days of more physical activity, from noon to 11 p. m. The temporal association was not explained by potential confounders such as morning pain, mood or effects of the circadian rhythm."

The more sleep chronic pain sufferers got at night, the more energy they had the next day, and thus the more physical activity they engaged in.

Why is that important? Because many who suffer chronic pain do not have the energy to engage in physical activity (even walking, grocery shopping, house cleaning and other seemingly-simple things).

GETTING BETTER SLEEP

I have written several articles at www.easyhealthoptions.com on how to get a better night's sleep and overcome insomnia. The essentials to a better night sleep are:

- Go to bed at the same time every night.
- Wake up at the same time every morning.
- Do not eat within three hours of bedtime.
- Do not consume alcohol or caffeine within six hours of bedtime.

- Create a comfortable, dark and quiet sleeping environment.
- Don't read in bed, especially from a backlit eReader.

That last point is a new problem with a direct effect on sleep quantity and quality.

EREADERS – THE HIDDEN SLEEP WRECKERS

Well, with all new inventions comes a period of time before people notice changes in their health. And when the number of complaints reaches critical mass, someone conducts a study. Luckily for us, a new study by the Proceedings of the National Academy of Sciences of the United States of America looked into the negative effects of the "evening use of light-emitting eReaders and how they negatively affect sleep, circadian timing and next-morning alertness."

The researchers found that when people use eReaders before bedtime, there are several very clear side effects:

- It takes longer to fall asleep.
- It delays the circadian clock.
- It suppresses levels of the sleep-promoting hormone melatonin.
- It delays the timing of REM sleep.
- It reduces alertness the following morning.

The reason for these adverse effects is that these devices increase alertness at bedtime, even more so than reading a printed book (which also is not recommended for insomniacs). Being more alert means it's more difficult to fall into sleep. According to researchers:

"This negative impact on sleep may be due to the short-wavelength enriched light emitted by these electronic devices, given that artificial-light exposure has been shown experimentally to produce alerting effects, suppress melatonin and phase-shift the biological clock."

As a chronic pain sufferer myself, I know it is easy to say, "just get more sleep and you will have less pain and derive more energy."

Yet, pain is what keeps many sufferers from sleeping deeply at all, let alone through the night. It's a vicious cycle, a catch 22: Sleep provides more energy for physical activity; and physical activity reduces pain; but pain prevents sleep.

All we can do is understand the pain-sleep connection, know that it is real and take steps to improve sleep by avoiding eReaders, caffeine, food, exercise and other things at night that keep us alert – and do this enough to create a new habit that will allow us to fall asleep more easily and for longer duration. In the mornings, we'll feel better and have more energy to do more physical things.

REFERENCES:

http://www.ncbi.nlm.nih.gov/pmc/articles/PMC3880190/

http://www.painmed.org/patientcenter/facts_on_pain.aspx#highlights

http://www.cdc.gov/features/dssleep/

http://journals.plos.org/plosone/article?id=10.1371/journal.pone.0092158

http://www.pnas.org/content/early/2014/12/18/1418490112.abstract

http://easyhealthoptions.com/get-best-sleep-ever/

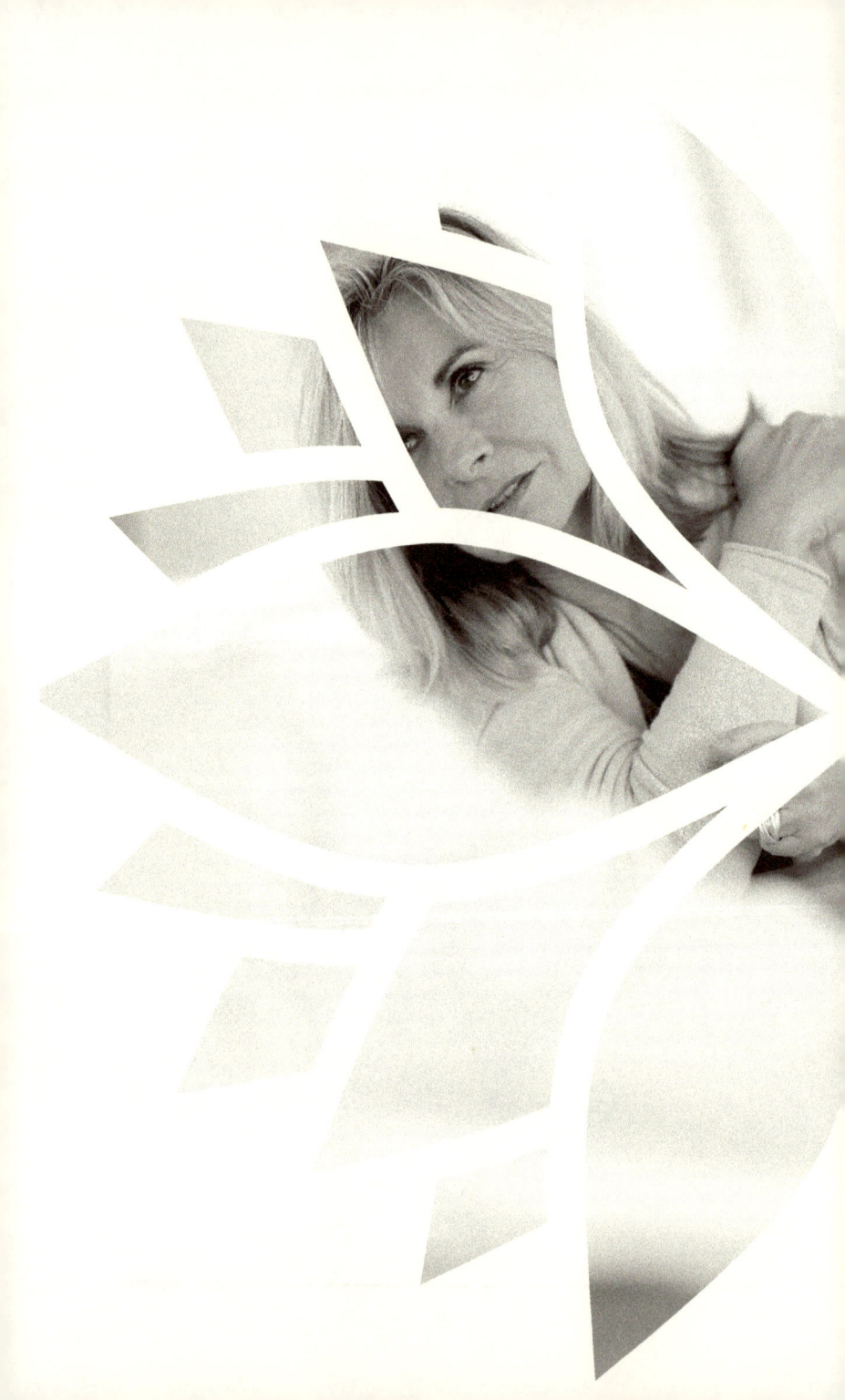

CHAPTER 4

THE FIBROMYALGIA PUZZLE – PAIN RELIEF STARTING TODAY

Pain is the debilitating bane of our lives. It comes in all shapes and sizes and at various times and places. Sometimes, the reason for pain is identifiable; at other times, it is not so easily pinpointed.

The conventional medical establishment, unable to explain the precise reasons people feel pain in multiple places, coined the term fibromyalgia. With this term, it neatly categorized a whole spectrum of pain under a single disease label.

FIBROMYALGIA, THE NEW DISEASE

Fibromyalgia is a chronic pain syndrome that still eludes specific definition. One of the key symptoms is extreme pain in multiple areas of the body, wherein there is tenderness to light touch. Add to this – fatigue, digestive issues, disruption of sleep and cognitive impairment, and the issues get a bit complicated.

Theories of links to viruses and infections, emotional disorders associated with decreased opioid receptor activity and physical trauma are abundant. Some posit fibromyalgia as the body's reaction to stress or its abnormal response to it. And like classic migraine sufferers, those with fibromyalgia are sensitive to sounds, an indication of a possible abnormality in sensory processing by the central nervous system.

The problem with fibromyalgia is that it is debilitating and restrictive. Pain tires not only the body, but also the mind and spirit. It deflates your mood, ruins sleep, derails work and blocks the experience of life's joys. Too much pain causes people to take medications and pills to kill the throbbing, dull the aching, reduce the inflammation and loosen the spasm. These are fine for short-term relief; but over the long haul, they do more harm to the body than good.

Natural solutions are best, and there are plenty.

ROOT CAUSE

Experts admit they don't know the root cause of fibromyalgia. And since it is a term applied to non-specific chronic pain at different locations on the body, it is hard to pin down.

If we forget the label applied to this disorder for a moment and instead focus on its symptoms, we see pain, an imbalanced nervous system, insomnia and a disquieted mind, leading to low mood. Chinese medicine and other natural wellness perspectives view these as symptoms of several imbalances, like sluggish blood flow, hyperactivity of the nerves and emotional trauma. If each of these symptoms is addressed naturally, then the overall symptoms and continuity of chronic pain decrease.

Let's look at ways to treat these problems:

Exercise: Yes, exercising when in pain may seem counterintuitive. When you're in pain, especially chronic pain, it is difficult to even think about exercising. But there are exercises that are gentle, like slow walking, yoga, tai chi, qigong and stretching. When dealing with body pain, moving the body is essential.

Movement helps maintain range of motion that shortens from lack of use. Those tight shoulders and hips that make you strain when retrieving the plate from the cabinet or getting into and out of the car feel a whole lot better if range of motion is restored or normalized. Walking or waving the arms moves fresh blood, oxygen and nutrients throughout the body. It also makes you sweat, releasing toxins that otherwise stagnate and cause pain. And movement prevents connective tissue from adhering and "gluing" muscles together, like scar tissue.

Getting up and moving, even slowly and gently at first, should be the first step for decreasing pain and removing the symptoms of chronic pain and/or fibromyalgia.

Water aerobics are often especially useful. Research from Spain has shown that patients who engage in water aerobics are able to reduce fibromyalgia pain. The study consisted of 33 women diagnosed with fibromyalgia between the ages of 37 to 71. It found that water exercise "enhances the health-related quality of life in women with fibromyalgia." Water aerobics is a form of low-impact exercise that should be considered a viable alternative to walking or yoga if these prove too painful at the start.

Meditation: The benefits of mediation have been documented in dozens of studies. Meditation has been shown to lower blood pressure, which can help decrease pain. It relaxes the central nervous system, which helps decrease pain. It slows breathing and the thought process, which helps clear mental and emotional issues to help ease pain. And it relaxes the body to induce sleep. It is in deep sleep that the body relaxes and repairs, which is needed to reduce and prevent pain and inflammation.

Anti-inflammatory Diet: Diet plays a major role in pain and fibromyalgia. It is important for those with chronic pain to avoid too much sugar, fats, trans fats, acidic foods, hydrogenated oils and dairy. In turn, it is best to increase foods high in fiber, omega-3 fatty acids and antioxidants. These include fruits, vegetables (especially the green leafy variety) and whole grains (especially oats).

Supplements: There are several supplements that naturally help reduce inflammation and pain while elevating mood. These include:

- Omega-3 fats: high in the fatty acids DHA and EPA, which help reduce inflammation and acidity, thus reducing pain.
- Turmeric: contains curcumin (its active component); helps reduce inflammation and pain.
- Feverfew: reduces vasoconstriction to normalize blood flow and reduce pain especially that associated with classic migraine.
- Arnica: topical cream that helps reduce pain and inflammation.
- St. John's wort: has been shown to help with emotional disorders like depression (a cause and symptom of pain).
- Chamomile: helps relax the mind at night before bed, which can reduce stress-induced insomnia.
- Other Chinese and Indian herbal formulas for pain: best used under the guidance of a practitioner after a physical examination.

When all is considered, we have the power to control this pain ourselves with our daily actions, habits and activities. Taking a proactive and focused role in your own pain management allows for natural reduction and prevention.

Simple changes in diet, physical activity, sleep, meditation and supplements can go a long way to helping you overcome this debilitating issue.

EXERCISE TO BOOST ENERGY AND BRAIN HEALTH – AND BANISH FIBROMYALGIA PAIN

Chronic pain conditions take their toll in many ways. Not only is there discomfort and suffering, but there is also a shift away from joy and happiness to depression and loss of will.

When one is in pain it is difficult to get up and move. The mind says yes but the body says no – until eventually the mind also says no.

The key is to stop this cycle and make a change.

Did you know that your body needs to expend energy to make energy? And that the more energy you make this way, the better you feel, physically and mentally? You have to get up and move to realize that doing so will clear the mental fog and also help your body feel better by reducing pain. Seems counterintuitive, but it's true.

This is why exercise is good for the body and it makes you feel good even after you're done. It is one of the healthiest things you can do for yourself, and as it turns out, exercise is not just for "getting fit" or "losing weight." A series of studies show that exercise helps improve mental health as well as how you perceive and handle pain. For chronic pain sufferers, this is vital because the pain/depression cycle is a tough one to overcome.

And with continuous pain there is a loss of quality of life because many things that once were enjoyable become chore-like; even simple things like riding a bike, gardening or taking a walk. And when the body is not moving, blood and endorphins (feel-good chemicals) are not actively surging through the body, bringing nutrients to muscles and euphoric feelings to the mind. And it's a vicious cycle because the more you hurt, the less you want to do, and the less you do the more depressed you become.

But you can reverse all of that and get stronger and more energetic as you age.

Let's review a few studies that shed light on how this can work for you.

CIRCULATION IMPROVES YOUR BRAIN

Researchers from the Norwegian University of Science and Technology at St. Olav University Hospital conducted a population-based cross-sectional study to assess how frequency, duration and intensity of physical activity were related to health-related quality of life. They looked at 4,500 participants (56% females and 44% males).

The study found that exercising, at any level, is associated with better physical and mental health in both genders compared with no exercise, particularly among the older individuals.

"I'M FEELIN' NO PAIN..."

According to a study carried out by researchers at the University of New South Wales and Neuroscience Research Australia, as one exercises more vigorously or for prolonged periods, the body adjusts to the discomfort in a positive way. The longer the workout the greater our ability to tolerate the pain and discomfort felt in the muscles. This happens through the body's natural release of adrenalin and endorphins, or feel-good chemicals, that weaken our awareness of, or increases our toleration for, discomfort. It is a phenomenon known as hypoalgesia.

To better understand the hypoalgesic effect, the researchers set out to examine the effect of aerobic exercise training on pain sensitivity in 24 healthy individuals over a six-week time frame. During this time participants cycled three times per week for 30 minutes at a time, at a measure of 75% of maximal oxygen usage. Researchers then measured the participant's blood pressure, pain threshold and tolerance by affixing and inflating a blood pressure cuff around their arms.

The results showed significant increases in aerobic fitness and pain tolerance after training. Conversely, the no-exercise control group showed no change in their physical fitness levels or in their pain threshold levels.

This led researchers to conclude that, *"Moderate-to vigorous-intensity aerobic exercise training increases ischemic pain tolerance in healthy individuals."*

In other words, people who exercised developed increased tolerance to pain while also becoming more fit.

EXERCISE REDUCES PAIN IN WOMEN WITH FIBROMYALGIA

A Spanish study published in the journal *Arthritis Care & Research,* looked at the association between fitness levels and pain levels in 468 women with fibromyalgia. The study hoped to characterize the association of different components of physical fitness with pain levels, pain-related catastrophizing and chronic pain self-efficacy. In other words, how fitness levels affect pain levels and how this affects one's negative view of future events.

What the researchers found was good news indeed. A higher level of fitness was consistently associated with a lower pain level experience, lower pain-related catastrophizing and increased ability to believe they can do things on their own. Those with higher combined muscle strength with flexibility experienced the lowest levels of pain.

These studies are important because they show scientifically what many in the wellness field have always known. The more you exercise the better you feel, physically and mentally. The more you do physically, the more you believe you are capable of. And the more you can do, the better your body adjusts to the effort, and the less pain you feel. And with less pain comes the ability and desire to do more. And with this comes less depression and a better overall quality of life. This is a cycle you want to be in!

FIBROMYALGIA RELIEF IN DAILY QIGONG PRACTICE

In the old days – say 5,000 years ago – the Chinese knew something very important: Reduce stress and tension in the body or become feeble and suffer in pain. To do this, they experimented with herbs and needles and meditative movements in the hopes of establishing and maintaining their quality of life.

They found that by slowing down, moving in a relaxed manner, regulating their breath and focusing their intention all at the same time, they could produce a systemic effect on the body that promoted wellness. That method is called qigong, and recent research has found it effective in relieving the leading symptoms of fibromyalgia.

Because fibromyalgia is a syndrome, and not a disease, it is better to adjust the body systemically in a natural and gentle way, than to create more pain and side effects with pain medication and the like. But how to do that when pain relief in the moment is what patients want?

Ancient Chinese qigong practices may be the way.

QIGONG, THE BASICS

Qigong means *breath work*, or *breath cultivation*. But more than that it refers to slowing the breath and focusing the intention to build qi, or *internal energy*. There are many schools of qigong falling into categories of medical, religious and martial, but all work from the same premise even though their specifics and goals maybe different.

The fundamental practice of qigong involves four things:

1) Posture (standing, seated, lying);
2) Breath regulation (with chest or abdominal expansion and counting);
3) Movement (of one or more body parts); and
4) Intention (focusing the mind). The Chinese have a saying that the mind/intention leads the qi/energy. And so one cannot cultivate their qi (energy) if the mind (intention) is not focused on the breath, the posture and the movement.

All of these four areas must be in sync for the best results. In other words, if moving the hands apart slowly, the movement must be slow and purposeful, the mind focused on the task and the space between the hands, and the breath must start and stop when the hand movement starts and stops.

When done altogether, changes occur in the body – most notably, relaxation and a quieting of the mental chatter that stresses people. From this practice, over time, comes a more supple musculature, less tension and trigger points in the muscles, less obstruction to the flow of blood, lymph and other body fluids and an overall feeling of lightness and wellbeing. Often times, along with these things people find a renewed energy they forgot they had once possessed.

Recent research published in the journal, *Evidence-Based Complementary and Alternative Medicine*, looked at the positive effects of daily qigong practice on the main symptoms of fibromyalgia.

FIBROMYALGIA AND QIGONG

The authors of the new review article tell how in the mainstream medical and scientific literature, qigong is thought of and labeled as a "meditative movement," a "mindful exercise" and a "complementary exercise" that is being explored in terms of its potential impact on relieving the symptoms associated with fibromyalgia. Their approach to culling data was to do a meta-analysis and summarize the results of randomized controlled trials (RCT) and other studies on qigong published up through the end of 2013.

The results were positive and indicate that *"regular qigong practice (daily, six to eight weeks) produces improvements in core domains for fibromyalgia (pain, sleep, impact and physical and mental function) that are maintained at four to six months compared to wait-list subjects or baselines."*

CONCLUSION

In addition to helping reduce the symptoms of fibromyalgia, the researchers had this to say about the ancient Chinese practice:

"Some recent intriguing studies demonstrate that extended qigong practice can lead to changes at a molecular level. Thus, there is a report that extensive qigong practice (one to two hours daily, for at least a year) leads to altered expression of 250 genes in neutrophils compared to healthy controls, with changes characterized by enhanced immunity, down-regulation of cellular metabolism and alteration in apoptotic genes in favor of resolution of inflammation."

Not too shabby, and certainly worth doing daily for a period of time to see how qigong practice can make you feel overall. As the researchers noted, the length of daily practice for an extended period showed the greatest results. So don't just try qigong... make it a part of your wellness lifestyle.

BEYOND FIBRO: SOOTHE NERVE PAIN NATURALLY

What do certain types of headaches, neck pain, back pain, fibromyalgia and sciatica have in common? They all share a common root cause of their pain: overactive nerves. The good news is that there are plenty of natural ways to reduce nerve pain; and research reveals a remarkable, counterintuitive method that offers effective relief.

Neuropathic pain, or nerve pain, is a common ailment that afflicts most of us at some point in our lives, and many people suffer from it chronically. While NSAIDs (nonsteroidal anti-inflammatory drugs) and prescription medications seem to be the first line pain-reduction used by many people because of their fast-acting strength, their side effects leave much to be desired.

COMMON CAUSES OF NERVE PAIN

Neuropathy is a painful condition that affects the peripheral nervous system, which includes the sensory, motor and autonomic nerves. These are the nerves related to the organs (including the skin) and muscles. When the nerves become dysfunctional through injury, disease or other conditions, you may experience numbness or tingling in the fingers and/or toes. Often, this pain can worsen and change into a burning sensation.

When it results from physical trauma or injury, the cause of nerve damage or nerve-related pain is easy to identify. However, even after an injury is believed to be healed, nerve damage can remain and the nerves don't return to their normal functioning state. In other cases, the root cause of the nerve problem remains unknown.

That's because not all causes of nerve pain are fully understood. And medical treatments are generally focused on toxic drug therapy. But there are natural, low-cost options available. Talk to your physician about these options, and make an information-gathering appointment with a local chiropractor, massage therapist, acupuncturist, herbalist or nutritionist to find out his experience in working with neuropathic pain. I am always a fan of taking the natural route when possible.

NATURAL RELIEF

Generally, neuropathic pain results when nerve signals from the spinal cord that go out to the body are disrupted. The key to prevention and relief is to clear the obstruction or the reason for the nerve-signal disruption.

When considering natural approaches to relieving nerve pain, consider the role of essential nutrients, herbal supplements, exercise and bodywork.

BODYWORK THERAPY

Since the basis of nerve pain is related to blockage of the nerve signal from the spinal cord to the sensory nerves of the body, correcting spinal and muscular imbalances is a good place to begin, including chiropractic and massage therapy.

Chiropractic, which is well-known in the United States, works effectively for neuropathic pain because of its focus on the spine. According to the theories of chiropractic, when the vertebrae of the spine are misaligned, they create nerve irritation or spasms along the paraspinal muscles that can compress the nerves of the spinal cord. These nerves, if irritated or compressed, are unable to send and receive proper signals from the muscles and sensory organs back to the brain for proper analysis.

When nerve function falters, symptoms include muscle spasms, trigger points, peripheral neuropathy, sciatica, numbness, tingling and burning pain.

A chiropractor palpates your spine to find where there is joint dysfunction and nerve impingement (subluxations). Then he applies specific spinal adjustments that correct these by returning the spine back to its normal functioning state.

Massage therapists, while not aligning the spine with a manual adjustment, help in other ways. Massage helps relieve muscle spasm and inflammation by removing stagnations of body fluids like blood and lymph, and helping return normal movement in dysfunctional muscles and tissues. Massage therapy can relieve the spasms in the back, neck, shoulders and hips that can pull the spine to one side or compress or irritate the nerves coming from the spine. This relaxation and improved blood flow helps reduce neuropathic pain by correcting some of its causes. A combination of massage and chiropractic is a good choice for pain relief.

NUTRIENTS AND SUPPLEMENTS

Another cause of nerve pain is deficiency of some essential nutrients, especially magnesium. According to *The Journal of Physiology*, magnesium decreases nerve pain by calming the neurotransmitter NMDA. Overstimulation of this brain chemical is a known cause of nerve pain; magnesium has been shown to calm it without side effects. There are several forms of magnesium on the market, but the chelated form at 500 mg per day has shown strong absorption and alleviation for nerve pain, headaches and muscle spasms.

Devil's Claw (harpagophytum) and Burdock (Arctium lappa) have known anti-inflammatory properties, as do vitamin D3 and curcumin (turmuric). German chamomile (Matricaria recutita) and the Zanthoxylums (toothache tree and Hercules' club) have anti-inflammatory and anti-spasmodic properties. Reducing spasms and inflammation are two good ways to prevent and reduce nerve pain naturally.

ZAP YOUR PAIN AWAY WITH FSM THERAPY

Science has shown your body is "the body electric," made up of waves, particles, protons, electrons and atoms whirling around at tremendous speeds. In essence, we are electric, vibrating beings. Healing modalities like acupuncture, quantum touch, ultrasound and TENS units can have positive effects on your levels of pain and sense of well-being. But there is a relatively new treatment you should know about that's called frequency specific microcurrent (FSM) therapy. It uses low electric currents to heal bone and block pain.

WHAT IS FSM?

FSM therapy specifically treats myofascial pain by reducing inflammatory cytokines (polypeptide regulators). In other words, it helps reduce trigger points and connective tissue constrictions that cause pain and other sensations, like "pins and needles," coldness or burning, and numbness or itching caused by a damaged or diseased sensory system.

FSM is a noninvasive therapy that requires the use of a two-channel microamperage current device operated by a trained practitioner. The treatment requires two separate channels of voltage to be connected to the patient while he attempts to move his affected limbs to their utmost range of motion. Clinical studies show that the specific frequency combination of 13Hz and 396Hz, when used simultaneously, can effectively treat nerve and muscle pain, reduce inflammation and clear scar tissue. Other frequency combinations have been shown to reduce the pain associated with kidney stones and aid in healing of asthma, liver dysfunction, irritable bowel syndrome (IBS), shingles, low back pain, fibromyalgia and other conditions.

STUDIES SHOW PROMISE

While FSM therapy is relatively new, electric frequencies have been used for decades (although the less said about shock therapy, the better). In 1980, microcurrent technology was used by physicians in Europe and the United States for stimulating bone repair in nonunion fractures. There are numerous studies published on the effects of single-channel microcurrent showing that it increases the rate of healing in wounds and fractures.

A study published in the journal *Clinical Orthopaedics and Related Research* in 1982, showed that microamperage current between 10 and 500 micro amps increases ATP (cellular energy) production by 500% in rat skin. The article explains how, *"ATP is the chemical that the body uses for energy. The current also increased amino acid transport into the cell by 70% and waste product removal."* That's rather impressive.

The *Journal of Bodywork and Movement Therapies* published an article on the positive use of FSM to treat fibromyalgia patients. It is also an impressive showing of results for pain relief. Allow me to share some of the abstract with you here.

- Patients who have fibromyalgia syndrome (FMS) associated with cervical spine trauma have distinct pain descriptors and physical examination findings. Currently, there is no effective treatment for fibromyalgia.

- A total of 54 consecutive patients meeting the ACR diagnostic criteria for fibromyalgia were treated with micro-amperage current. Blood samples on a subset of six patients were analyzed using a recycling immune-affinity chromatography system to identify objective changes accompanying subjective pain scores.
- Five patients did not tolerate treatment. The remaining 49 patients reported reduction in pain on a 10-point visual analog scale (VAS) from an average baseline score of 7.37±1.2 to 1.37±1.1 with the first treatment.
- Thirty-one patients reported symptomatic relief from fibromyalgia following an average of eight treatments.
- Median time to improvement was 2 months and the actuarial recovery curve reached 100% at 4.5 months.
- The subjective outcomes scores in conjunction with biological markers for pain and pro-inflammatory cytokines observed in response to this treatment protocol are important preliminary findings.

FSM is successful, I believe, because it uses microcurrent electrical signals. These are at the same frequency as our cells, which is important because when higher frequencies are used, the nervous system is activated and can be counterproductive. TENS units work at higher frequencies and are less successful at pain reduction that the FSM (as shown in research). More than just a pain blocker, FSM therapy seems to adjust our biological system to increase ATP production, amino acid transport and waste product removal from cells. This combination reduces inflammation and pain as a result of real changes, not just blocked nerve pathways.

FSM is said to help many types of pain, from shingles to back pain to fibromyalgia. If you have tried just about everything and are still in pain, perhaps looking into this therapy may offer some relief.

ENERGY AND EXERCISE

Increasing your energy can also prevent and relieve neuropathic pain naturally. Acupuncture helps via the insertion of fine filaments (needles) into the skin along meridians or energy channels at specific points. The needles act as antennae that draw in bioelectric energy into the body to normalize energy, blood flow and nerve signals by correcting energetic imbalances that affect these areas.

Physical exercise is another natural and no-cost way to relieve nerve pain. It seems counterintuitive since most people in pain do not want to exercise. However, a study in the June 2012 issue of the journal *Anesthesia & Analgesia* reports that exercise appears to reduce neuropathic pain by a whopping 30-50% by reducing levels of inflammation-causing substances called cytokines. It turns out that exercise boosts levels of a protein called HSP27 (heat shock protein-27), which is believed to reduce cytokine levels that cause inflammation and, thus, nerve pain.

REFERENCES:

http://www.ncbi.nlm.nih.gov/pubmed/21131869
http://www.ncbi.nlm.nih.gov/pubmed/24504426
http://onlinelibrary.wiley.com/doi/10.1002/acr.22610/abstract
http://www.hindawi.com/journals/ecam/2014/379715/
http://easyhealthoptions.com/natural-relief-for-fibromyalgia-pain/
http://www.frequencyspecific.com/papers.php
http://healthdocs.org/?p=59&option=com_wordpress&Itemid=86

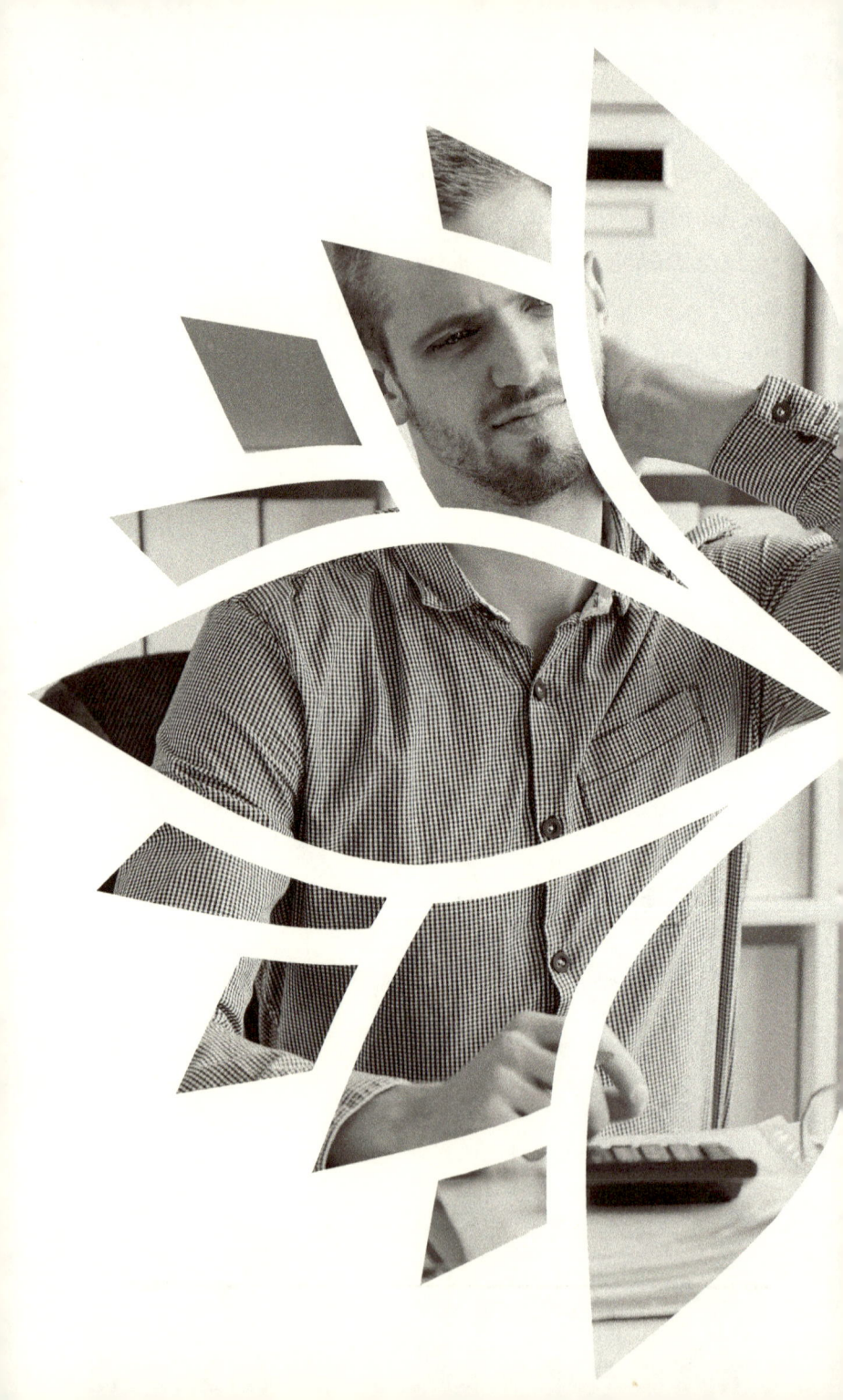

CHAPTER 5

WHAT TO DO ABOUT YOUR PAIN IN THE NECK

*N*eck pain is one of those wellbeing issues that can really interfere with your life. But whether you're hurt or you just woke up with a stiff neck, here's what you can do...

Psychological stress, poor sleep habits, bad posture, physical trauma, sports strain and age-related ailments can all cause various forms of issues that result in neck pain. What's more, the pain in the neck usually affects the shoulders, arms and hands by causing tightening, weakness, shooting pain and limited range of motion.

Gaining an understanding of the mechanisms of neck pain is just as important for moving toward relief as is the correct treatment method itself. It is difficult to maintain a quality of life when you have a pain in the neck.

NECK PAIN BASICS

Although 10% of Americans suffer from neck pain annually, there really is no way to prevent it. In fact, there are many causes of neck pain, some more serious than others. But the good news is that most neck pain is not the result of some serious illness. In fact, like back pain, neck pain comes and goes with the normal ebb and tide of life. For many people, it lasts only a week or two in most cases. In more serious cases it can last for eight weeks.

THE STRUCTURE OF NECK PAIN

The Skeletal System is the scaffolding of the human body. It creates a structure and support for your body to be in its normal state. However, when the bones of the neck (cervical vertebrae) becomes diseased, out of alignment or compressed, pain can be the result. This happens by negatively affecting the discs between the bones, the muscles around them and thus the functioning of the nerve that runs through them.

The Muscular System is the mode of movement of the body. Contracting, flexing and extending muscles allow the body to move here and there, turn and twist and grasp. When the muscles around the neck and shoulders become tight in spasm, they make it difficult to turn or bend the neck. This limited range of motion can cause discomfort, pain and a compression of the vertebrae and potentially the nerves.

Intervertebral Discs are the gel-like material that rests between the neck bones, cushioning them and creating a nice space for the nerves to move through and out of the cervical vertebrae. However, when the discs become herniated or protrude, they restrict the space through which the nerves exist causing compression and pain.

The Nerves themselves are the cables that carry the signals from the brain to the rest of the body. They tell the organs and nervous system how to operate. They let us know when we feel pain, and when irritated or compressed, they can cause great pain that radiates from the neck to the shoulders, arms and down to the fingers.

Neck pain that is not related to serious issues, like infection or a tumor, is usually related to a combination of the conditions mentioned above. Before getting into some of the treatment options, let's take a look at some of the most common causes and symptoms of neck pain.

CAUSES AND SYMPTOMS OF NECK PAIN

Osteoarthritis is caused by a narrowing of the cartilage between the neck bones causing bone spurs leading to pain in the neck and referred pain to the arms.

Muscle Strain is caused by repetitive motion through a prolonged activity, like typing on the computer, creative work with the hands like painting, sculpting or plumbing. Muscle strain also comes from poor posture while sleeping or sitting, wherein the head is held for extended periods in a compromised position.

Whiplash and Stingers are basically the same issue, wherein the neck pain is caused from trauma to the soft tissue of the neck. Rear-end car accidents cause a whipping of the neck forward and backward, and athletes in sports like wrestling and football also experience a similar event through their physical contact with another person.

Forward Head Posture is the result of the head being held forward of the shoulders. This causes the muscles of the shoulders and neck to have to tighten more than normal to keep the head from falling more forward and bring you off balance.

Disc Herniation is a more serious issue that can cause numbness or tingling in the hands, loss of strength and acute pain. When the discs rupture or bulge they put pressure on the nerves that travel down the arm and in severe cases can also affect the function of the bladder.

Spinal Stenosis is when there is a narrowing of the spinal canal. Although this is more common with age, it causes a compression of the spinal cord through a thickening of the spinal ligaments and bone spurs, leading to neck pain and referred hand pain, weakness and numbness.

Wrong Sleeping Posture. Waking up with a stiff and painful neck is quite common. Many people do not know that a sleeping position, the posture of your body, actually affects your state of well-being.

The worst posture is stomach sleeping. It provides little support for the low back, and the shoulders press into the neck as the head is turned to either side. Sleeping with one or both arms above the head or under the pillow also causes neck strain and cramping because the raised arms press the scapula and scapular muscles up toward the head and affect the neck. The best posture is side sleeping with arms held at chest height, like the fetal position. If wrong sleeping posture is the cause of your acute or chronic neck pain, it is easily fixed by mindfully changing your posture. It may take a few days to relax, but it will happen.

Stress. Dealing with and repressing the stress of daily life is an undeniable factor in neck and low back pain. Physical, emotional and psychological stress comes from sources like work, family and friends. The mind's inability to deal with such stressors allows negative effects and damages cells. It slows the blood flow, cramps muscles and results in chronic pain. When stress leads to shallow breathing, tightens muscles and restricts blood flow, it causes oxygen deprivation. Working through stress helps reduce and prevent chronic pain. There are many therapies available for stress reduction, including biofeedback, meditation, yoga, tai chi, qigong, massage and acupuncture. The best route is one that not only helps reduce pain in the immediate moment but also shuts it down at the source by influencing the mind. If stress is an issue in your neck pain, meditation can play a key role in its control, as well as methods like neuro-linguistic programming (NLP), the Sedona Method, eye movement desensitization and reprocessing (EMDR), emotional freedom technique (EFT) and, often, relieving tension myositis syndrome (TMS).

Spinal Subluxation. This refers to disorders of the spine that display a shift in vertebral alignment. Herniated discs, muscle imbalances and natural changes in the spine can cause the spine to become misaligned (subluxated). Commonly, this is caused by poor posture that is maintained for days, weeks or months. This may occur throughout your lifetime. Sitting hunched forward in the car or at the desk, carrying a backpack slung over one shoulder, poor sleeping posture or standing with weight on one leg all can cause a shift in the natural alignment of the hips, spine and body overall. This causes strain on certain muscle groups, pulls on the spinal column and may irritate or impinge on nerves to cause pain. Treatment by a chiropractor or osteopathic physician trained in spinal adjustment techniques and by massage therapists who work on soft tissue and deep tissue, as well as attending yoga classes, will help correct the issue over time. However, being mindful to change your posture at each point along the day will do the most in terms of prevention.

Cervical Subluxation, or misalignment of the neck bones, can cause narrowing of the space where nerves reside. This creates irritation and pain that is localized and radiates. Subluxation can also cause the neck muscle to tighten in their way of protecting the body, which also causes spasm pain.

Energy Blockages. Changes in the energy of the body are not uncommon. This can happen through negative thought patterns, being exposed to electromagnetic fields (EMF) and poor diet. The idea of energy blockages is a common concept in acupuncture, where the body is seen as being influenced by dozens of energy channels (meridians) that need to be clear to avoid pain, illness and disease. Receiving acupuncture or acupressure along the meridians of the neck, shoulders and back can help alleviate neck stiffness and pain. But changing diet and thoughts and reducing stress will help prevent the issue from recurring in the organ systems that feed energy to the channels in those areas.

TREATMENT OPTIONS

While there are quite a few reasons for you to experience pain and discomfort in your neck, the actual results are quite similar. These include, as outlined above, vertebral misalignment, muscle spasm, disc disease and narrowing of the spinal canal. In cases of traumatic neck pain, you should consult a physician for tests to see if there is serious injury.

Here are some simple steps I advise, and that I take myself when experiencing pain.

Step 1. Consider what has transpired over the course of the days and hours leading up to your neck pain attack. If it is serious, like whiplash from an accident, be sure to seek medical examination and care. If it is not serious, move to step 2.

Step 2. Your neck pain may be caused by stress, sleeping wrong or shoulder tightness rather than a serious problem; you need to determine what the pain is associated with.

Each type of pain or cause should be addressed in a simple way that helps the issue. If no serious issue is at work, then each of these can be treated in the same way. Here are some examples.

- **Rest and Relaxation** is your best friend. By this, I don't mean sleeping your day away, but finding ways to reduce more physical strain and psychological stress. Learning to take it easy is important, and in addition to sleep, you can use self-hypnosis techniques, mediation and a cervical pillow to allow the muscles to feel no additional threat and thus relax. Massage is also quite useful for relaxing the mind, body and structures of the neck and shoulders.

- **Topical Analgesics** are a good way to reduce pain and inflammation by increasing blood flow to the affected area. They are generally safer and less toxic to the body than ingesting NSAIDs (nonsteroidal anti-inflammatory drugs), but they do tend to have a strong odor.

- **Chiropractic** adjustments are a good way to help return range of motion to the cervical vertebrae. If the chiropractor is skilled at palpating (feeling the neck with his hands), he can do an adjustment at the level of the subluxation.

- **Physical Therapy** is another good method for relief as it utilizes methods of strengthening the weaker neck structures while stretching the tighter ones to better bring balance back to the neck.

Other treatment options include acupuncture, traction devices, TENS units, muscle energy technique and the list goes on and on.

GETTING A HANDLE ON THE ISSUE

If you can see when or why it happens, then you can make changes to ensure neck pain becomes less frequent in your life. So if you wake up with a stiff neck, change your sleeping posture or pillows. If you neck hurts after sports, adjust what you are doing or its frequency. If your neck hurts by 3PM, then stress is the cause. You must find ways to reduce it.

Whether your neck pain is sudden with a direct onset of pain, or comes as a gradual worsening over time, your quality of life depends on getting a handle on it.

Once the cause of the stiffness or your pain has been determined (and there may be several causes), you must seek proper self-care and assisted care, and then stay on the path toward relief. Merely "trying" a therapy and not following it through will not do enough to alleviate a neck issue.

While working on the specific issues and receiving treatments where and when necessary, you can help reduce pain, stiffness and/or inflammation with supplements like curcumin and valerian.

Also helpful are hot baths and applications of heat and cold packs and rubs like Biofreeze® (made from herbal extracts) and Sombra® (a pain-relieving gel).

SCRAPING PAIN AWAY

Chronic pain and muscle spasms can put a serious cramp in your lifestyle. When it hurts to get out of bed, hurts to get dressed and hurts to carry out daily activities, life becomes torture. But a wonderful Chinese technique called *gua sha* can scrape away that pain and actually offer enough relief to make pain medications unnecessary.

A Form of Bodywork

Gua sha can be thought of as a form of bodywork. It is similar to massage, but is carried out with a blunt instrument. Also, it is only applied to one area at a time and in only one direction.

Let's say you experience tightness or a chronic trigger point in your shoulders. When you receive gua sha, you sit, shoulders exposed to the practitioner. The practitioner's fingers press along the line of your shoulder. If the fingers show white marks on your skin after being removed, this is considered to be a sign of blockage. The blood and fluids are not moving freely in the shoulder, and this is the cause of the pain. When the sha, or white compression marks, take a long time to disappear, the problem has been there for a long period of time or the trouble spot lies deep within the muscle.

After initially testing the spot, the therapists lubricates the area and uses the blunt end of an instrument (like an old coin, rounded metal bottle cap, a piece of jade or hard plastic) to scrape over the troubled area. The movement is always deep, slow and steady and in the same direction away from the spine. (In other cases, like mid-back pain, the movement is parallel to the spine, but not toward or on it). The instrument is held at about a 30-degree angle, and the motion is repeated again and again until discoloration of the skin occurs.

During this process, patients often become worried. But there's no need for alarm. What is happening is that the repetitive motion of the instrument brings the toxic, stagnant blood and fluids to the surface of the skin where the lymphatic system can clear it. At the same time, as the old, stagnant blood is removed from the muscle, fresh blood carrying fresh oxygen and nutrients is brought into the area to aid in healing. While the skin surface looks as if

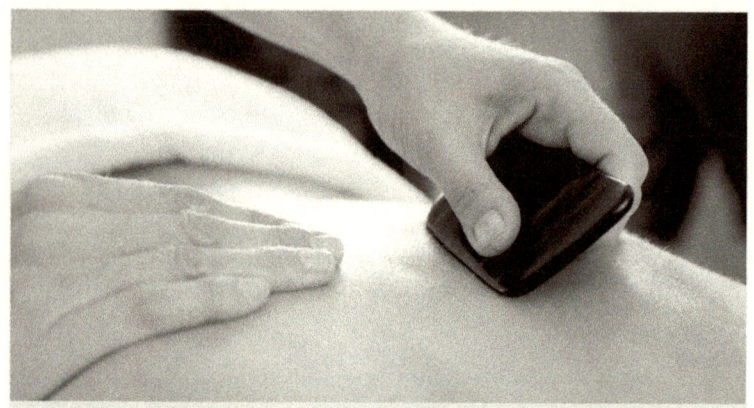

it is bruised, if the technique is performed properly, there should be no pain when the area is touched. This is a case where something looks worse than it feels. Interestingly, if there is no problem in that area, no dark discoloration comes to the surface and the skin retains its normal color.

Logical Treatment

While the 1,000-year-old method of gua sha may sound peculiar, it is actually based on the same logic used today in physical therapy and sports medicine. It is a form of deep-tissue massage or myofascial release. It augments soft-tissue mobilization. The process of applying the device gently, yet firmly, over the spasm area acts to mildly re-injure the area to promote proper healing.

In many cases, trigger points and muscle spasms are caused by injuries that may be decades old. These injuries often shorten muscles, tendons or ligaments after healing takes place improperly. Too much connective tissue can be formed which restricts movement and blood flow. Gua sha scraping breaks through this and allows for proper re-healing of the area, thereby correcting, once and for all, the origin of the pain and tightness.

While scraping can be performed on most muscles of the body, it should be avoided directly over bony areas, and never on a location where there is a new injury, painful bruising, sunburn, rash or break in the skin. Moles and pimples must be covered by the practitioner's fingers so they are not scraped and made painful.

The Very Idea

The very idea of scraping away pain, or causing a new micro-injury to heal an old chronic injury, and of allowing a practitioner to bring dark purple bruising to the surface of your skin may seem a little unreasonable and odd; but I'd like you to put aside your judgment of this ancient healing method and read more about it online. There are many sites, and pages and images available via a simple Internet search. If you can, call an acupuncturist or other bodywork therapist and ask if they are proficient in the method.

If so, give it a try. A few days of skin discoloration beats decades of pain meds and physical therapy.

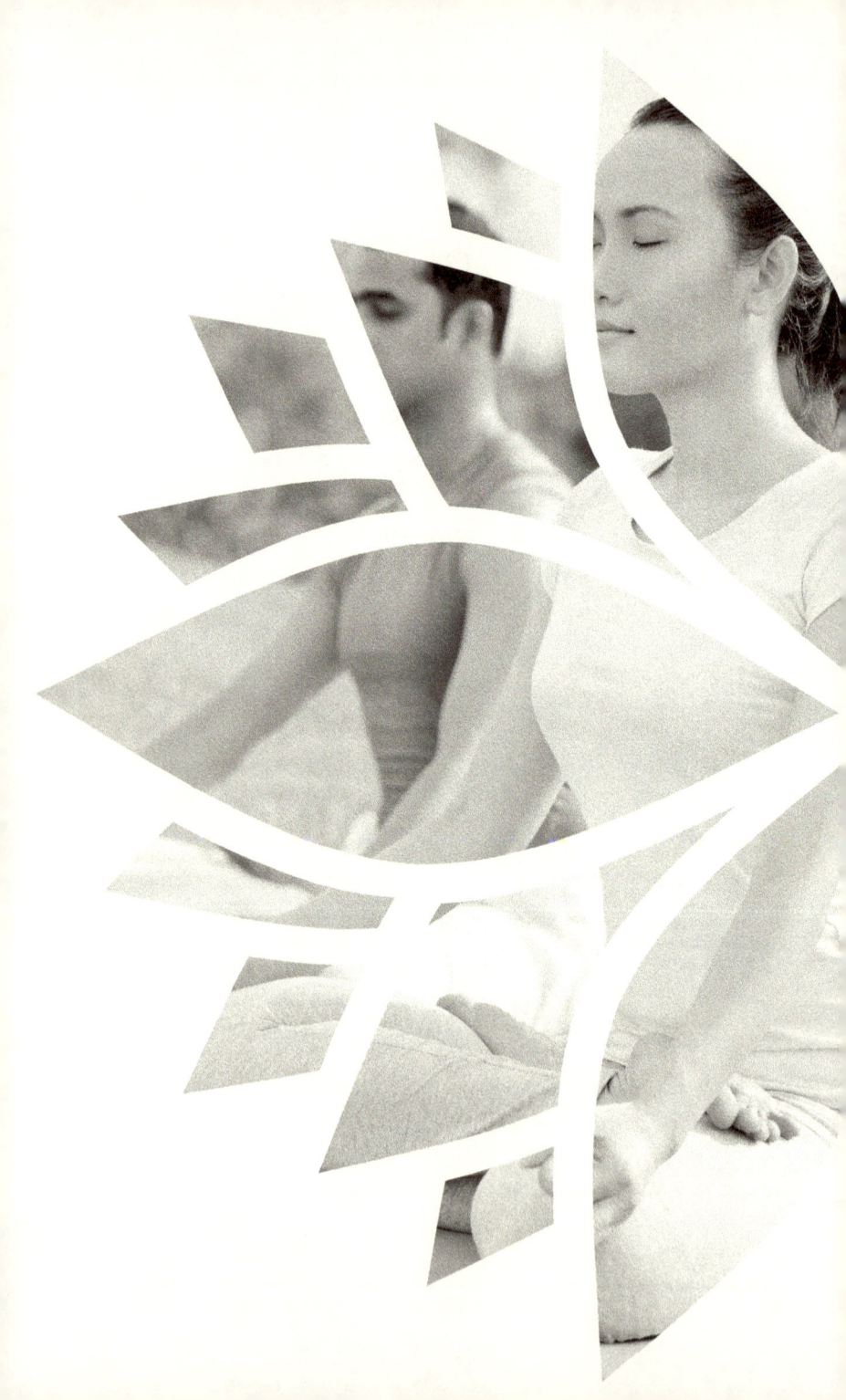

CHAPTER 6

SIX NATURAL WAYS TO REDUCE ACUTE PAIN AND MUSCLE SPASMS

Why are muscle spasms and pain so prevalent today when hundreds of hands-on therapies, over-the-counter medications and do-it-yourself techniques for pain reduction are available almost any time of day? The reason is not that the pills, pain patches and therapies don't work. Rather, the answer can most likely be found in your habits – known or unknown. The little things in your life, when combined day after day, can cause chronic muscle pain. Change those little things, and you can get big pain relief.

Muscle cramps and spasms become painful for a number of reasons. Most of the more serious reasons, like serious medical illness and traumatic injury, are less common and certainly need proper diagnosis and treatment. For many people suffering with chronic muscle pain, inflammation, cramps and spasms, the reasons are less serious. However, they are nonetheless vital to address in order to stop the pain-and-inflammation cycle and reduce the frequency, severity and duration of attacks.

If you experience daily muscle spasms or discomfort, the best thing you can do to help yourself is to get into a pattern of caring for yourself. In other words, be nice to yourself by not doing the things that can cause you more pain or discomfort and by doing the simple things that will help reduce and prevent a painful body. These six things are keys to lessening acute pain and spasms. Incorporating them into your daily life will help in many ways.

1. STAY HYDRATED WITH PLENTY OF PURE WATER

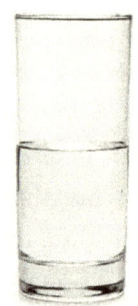

Water is one of the three essential things needed for life. (The others are oxygen and sunlight.) Water is so vital to life that life would not exist without it. While the human body is meant to be about 70% water, most people are chronically dehydrated. It is true that many people drink fluids throughout their day, yet they remain dehydrated. This happens when one consumes liquids that are diuretics.

Diuretics are substances that cause the body to excrete water. These include coffee, black tea, sodas and alcoholic beverages (particularly beer). When too many of these beverages are consumed, the body expels them quickly via urine and sweat. However, the body needs to retain enough purified fluids to maintain proper organ function, to remove toxins from the blood and to keep the skin moist. When water is low, toxins are not as easily processed or removed from the body and can begin recycling in the blood. This can cause pain, spasms and inflammation in the muscles.

Drinking eight to 10 glasses of purified or filtered water per day should bring you back to healthy levels within a few days. Some studies suggest people are habitually two quarts low of water.

Others demonstrate that as long as your urine is clear, then your water levels are good. Start with counting how many glasses of water you consume, then check your urine. You will feel the difference and discover the levels you need.

2. MAINTAIN YOUR MAGNESIUM LEVELS

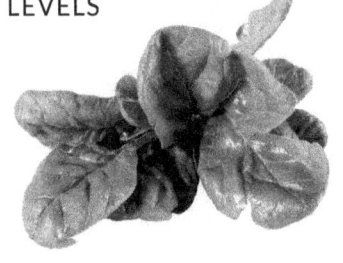

Magnesium is one of the essential minerals in the body that, when left unchecked, can lead to muscle spasms, cramping, pain and twitching. Magnesium helps all your organ systems function properly. Low levels of magnesium are a known cause of muscle pain. Most people need 300 mg to 400 mg of magnesium daily to help maintain proper functioning of the body. If supplementation is not your thing, then eating plenty of foods high in magnesium can do wonders. These include green leafy vegetables, whole grains and bran, soy beans and pumpkin.

Here's the scoop: Even if you get enough magnesium through diet or supplementation, your levels can still be decreased by internal causes. Irritable bowel syndrome (IBS), other gastrointestinal (GI) issues, diabetes, kidney disease or pancreatitis can be the cause of your decreased magnesium levels.

3. MAINTAIN YOUR POTASSIUM LEVELS

Like magnesium, potassium is essential to body function. When the body's magnesium levels are low, they can negatively impact potassium levels. When potassium levels drop below 3.7 mEq/L, the body has what is known as hypokalemia, which causes one to become weak and feel fatigued and causes muscles to twitch and cramp. This is because potassium is necessary for nerve signals, muscle contractions and fluid balance.

Potassium is best ingested in natural food forms. It is found in fruits (most notably apricots, bananas, raisins and figs), wheat bran, wheat germ, dried fruits, mixed seeds, beans and vegetables. Most common cereals and breads are fortified with this mineral. If you think low potassium may be a cause of your muscle pain and ailments, contact your local healthcare provider for the recommended blood screening.

4. EXERCISE AND STRETCH EVERY DAY

Exercise is another simple thing that you can do every day to become healthier and prevent needless pain and inflammation.

I know it is difficult to think about exercising when you are in pain. However, the main purpose of exercising for pain relief is to bolster blood flow. Even simple walking will help reduce your levels of muscle imbalances.

Walking for 30 minutes at an even pace, engaging in a simple stretching routine or participating in a yoga class will all help align the spine, keep the muscles supple and engender blood flow. When the blood is flowing well, a fresh supply of oxygen and nutrients move in the body, helping reduce pain and inflammation, repair the effects of stress and strain and move toxins out of the body. Think of muscle spasms as stagnations of blood trapped in the tissue and causing pain.

5. REDUCE STRESS WITH MIND-BODY TECHNIQUES

Do you rub your neck or low back constantly while at work or around certain people or events? This is stress making itself felt. Stress is a necessary part of life and of our survival. However, unhealthy stress can lead to excessive worry, anxiety, insomnia, improper breathing, muscle spasms and pain. While it is easy to suggest that you evaluate your life and remove all things and people that cause too much stress, this is not easily (or practically) done.

The good news is that there are quite a few simple mind-body techniques that can help reduce the effects and severity of stress. These include methods like biofeedback, mindful meditation, yoga, qigong, visualizations and hypnotherapy.

Looking into some of these and putting them into daily practice will go a long way to reducing the negative effects of stress on the body.

6. GET A GOOD NIGHT'S SLEEP

Sleeping well is another essential element the body needs in order to repair and rebuild.

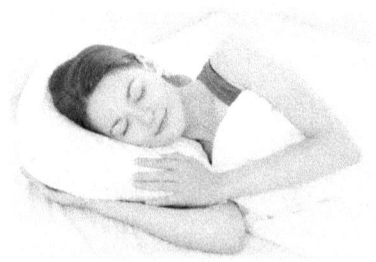

Even with a diet rich in magnesium and potassium, plenty of water and exercise and stress-reduction techniques, lack of ample deep sleep keeps the body from fully repairing itself. Sleeping at least seven hours in a position that will not cause you pain is necessary.

The secret to pain-free deep sleep is to set a standard sleep and wake-time cycle. Not reading or drinking before bedtime also helps reduce insomnia and waking to urinate during the night. Sleeping on your back or on your side with a pillow between the knees will keep the spine in a supported position to decrease chances of pinched nerves or muscle spasms from poor sleep posture. The key is to get into the habit of regular sleep that allows you to wake up feeling refreshed and ready for the day – not stiff, tired and anxious.

Yes, I have mentioned these 6 things before. But I mention them again as a list, to reinforce their importance to living a pain free life. To be sure, they will be mentioned again.

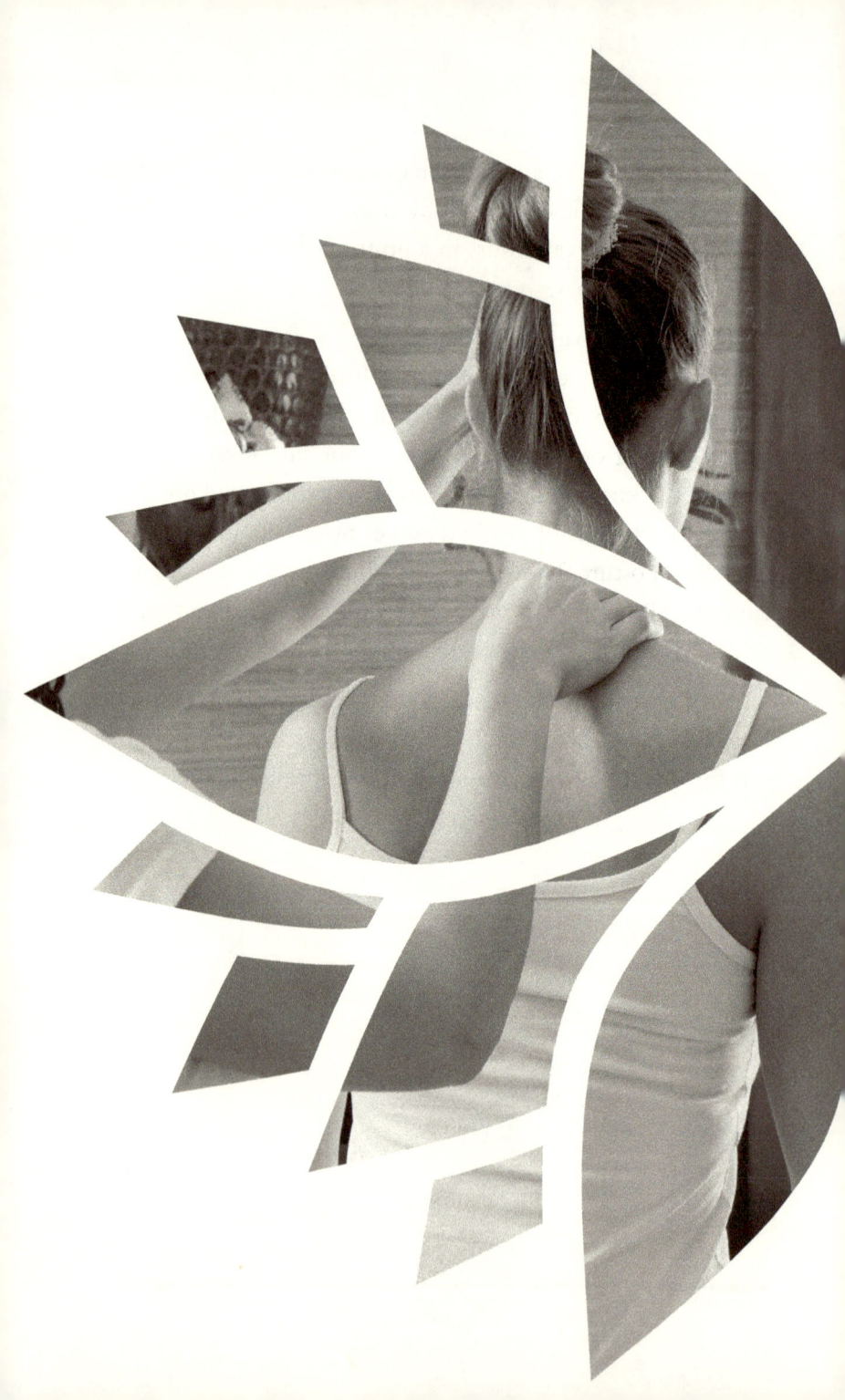

CHAPTER 7

NATURAL PAINKILLING SOLUTIONS

*I*t's an abomination: According to the Centers for Disease Control and Prevention (CDC), between the years 1999 and 2010, there was an enormous and unexpected rise in deaths from opioid pain-killers. Women fared much worse than men, with a 415% increase in deaths; men had a 265% increase in deaths.

Let's be clear: These are deaths of folks who were prescribed and took Food and Drug Administration-approved painkillers for pain conditions that could likely have been relieved by natural methods. So the deaths were needless and avoidable.

Specifically, 48,000 women were killed by these drugs. CDC Director Thomas Frieden said: *"Prescription painkiller drug deaths have skyrocketed in women… It is not only deaths, but there is also a great increase in the number of emergency department visits for misuse and abuse… of opioid painkillers."*

While the CDC states that such results could not have been indicated clinically, it ascertains that the larger number of deaths in women is indicative of the fact that more women than men experience chronic pain. Yet, despite protocol, the women have been getting higher doses of the painkillers than men, elevating their risk of death.

The scariest part is that physicians have been quick to prescribe high-level prescription painkillers for conditions for which they are not indicated. In other words, when it comes to opioids, they are indicated for cancer patients. There is no clear indication of their effectiveness and safety for noncancer-related pain therapy.

I will hand it to Frieden, though, as he made the accurate statement: *"These are risky drugs, and often there are other therapies such as physical therapy, exercise and cognitive therapies that can be important in addressing chronic pain."*

Here are a few recommendations I would like to make, and I hope that all people will consider them as the first line in their battle with acute and chronic pain.

TOPICAL CREAMS, GELS AND OILS FOR PAIN RELIEF

When searching for relief from pain, inflammation, swelling and stiffness, topical creams, gels and ointments can be quite effective. Topical pain products are mostly used for short-term relief. Once their active ingredients have metabolized in the body, their value is greatly diminished. For effectiveness over the long term (for chronic conditions), apply topical pain products three times per day as part of an overall program for arthritis relief.

Many of the most popular pain-relieving creams and gels share common ingredients. If you look at the product labels, you will likely see one or more of the following active ingredients, among others: Wintergreen, camphor, menthol, capsaicin and salicylate. Many of the most popular brands, like BENGAY®, Tiger Balm®, Mineral Ice® and so on share these ingredients.

Reaching for the common brands is OK, if that is all you have available. However, it is worth looking into some different brands that contain some ingredients you may not be familiar with, including: White Flower Analgesic Balm, Red Flower Oil, Po Sum On Medicated Oil, Wong Lop Kong Medicated Oil, Arnica Cream and Rub On Relief.

BODYWORK THERAPIES FOR PAIN RELIEF

Bodywork therapies are those that use the hands of a practitioner on your body to effect change in a positive way. Many who suffer with pain find it difficult to exercise because they are either too weak or in too much pain or because they have lost too much range of motion. In such cases, attending a series of hands-on bodywork sessions can really help loosen the body, align the system, free the nerves and awaken the energy. Here are some of the bodywork methods I find most helpful in diminishing pain and its somatic causes.

MASSAGE THERAPY

Massage improves circulation, and this is a big component of pain relief. A clear fluid called lymph circulates around our body's tissues. At the same time, you may have inflammation, which is an immune response to injury or infection that causes pain, redness, heat and swelling in the affected area. When lymph and inflammation start to accumulate in the body, the excess fluid puts pressure on blood vessels and circulation decreases, limiting blood flow. As the pressure increases, it irritates the nerves, which causes pain. By helping the body remove excess lymph and inflammation, massage therapy can assist with blood flow, which will reduce the pressure that is irritating the nerves and reduce your pain.

TRIGGER-POINT THERAPY

Trigger points are small contraction knots that develop in muscle and tissue when an area of the body is stressed, "frozen," injured or overworked. Sitting for too long a period of time or even restricting your movements can cause tiny land mines about the size of a dime to erupt deep in your muscle tissue. These are called trigger points; and they can occur in your back, arms, legs and feet. They are painful.

Deep and focused pressure to these areas can release this pain from your body. As the trigger point is compressed, your body will undergo soft-tissue release, allowing for increased blood flow, a reduction in muscle spasm and the breakup of scar tissue. It also helps remove any buildup of toxic metabolic waste. In other words, everything will again work the way it should.

THAI-YOGA MASSAGE

Thai-yoga massage is a gentle method of hands-on bodywork that is rhythmic and measured. The Thai-yoga therapist holds different body parts to gently stretch, press or compress them in a slow and rhythmic fashion that releases tension and fosters relaxation. Sometimes, the practitioner (who is usually a petite woman) will hold on to rails and use her feet and body weight to massage the back. The massage follows a sequence from head to toe. It releases the energy lines and connective tissue to induce a deep level of somatic correction and relaxation and to free up the body's range of motion.

NEED FOR RELIEF

Anyone suffering chronic pain needs relief. Your life is changed because of it in negative ways. Pain relief can come through natural means in safe and effective ways. There are many natural solutions to pain, such as diet, exercise, supplements, topical creams, bodywork therapies, energy medicine and cognitive therapies. Use these methods first before taking toxic prescription drugs. After all, you don't want to die trying to reduce your pain with prescription painkillers. You want to be pain-free to live and enjoy life.

THREE SUPER SPICES THAT KNOCK OUT PAIN

Here in the West, we think more in terms of nutritional supplements for health than we do food, let alone the flavorings we put into it. And we think even less of food as a pain reliever. Yet, flavor profiles like turmeric, capsaicin and ginger play a main role in pain relief.

Food, herbs and spices have been used for thousands of years for their powerful health-building and curative effects. Traditional cultures the world over have well developed medical systems based on substances that appear in nature.

Folk healing traditions of the Native Americans, Malaysians and Europeans all contain knowledge in the identification, procedures and uses of herbs.

Traditional Chinese medicine and Indian Ayurvedic medicine are among the oldest systems of medicine in the world, and they rely on herbals as a cornerstone of their practices.

The use of spices for healing is less well known, but those two traditions, traditional Chinese medicine (TCM) and Ayurveda, use mixtures of spices in their "food as medicine" principles, including relieving inflammation and pain.

Today, science has helped confirm that adding spices into your daily eating habits can go a long way toward low side effect, natural pain relief.

THE ROOT OF HEALTH, AND PAIN RELIEF

Turmeric is a brilliant yellow (and sometimes orange) root grated and used as one of the most recognizable flavorings in Indian cuisine. It's most active health-enhancing component is a substance called curcumin.

Curcumin is proven to reduce inflammation while helping the body to heal. Chronic, acute and low-grade inflammation are major causes of pain and poor health. While acute inflammation is a natural biological response to injury, stress and pathogens, its long-term effects are unhealthy, causing serious health concerns like heart disease.

The U. S. National Library of Medicine and the National Institutes of Health note: *"Laboratory and animal research has demonstrated anti-inflammatory, antioxidant and anti-cancer properties of turmeric and its constituent curcumin."*

Impressively, there are more than 5,500 peer-reviewed clinical studies demonstrating curcumin's benefits. Recent studies suggest that turmeric is as effective as, yet safer than, more than a dozen prescription medications. You can read about these benefits and their studies on pain, inflammation and cancer treatment in a few previous articles I've written at www.easyhealthoptions.com.

RED PEPPER PREVENTS PAIN?

Chili peppers, especially cayenne pepper, have a substance in them called capsaicin. Capsaicin is the part of the pepper that makes it hot and burns the tongue oh-so-nicely in spicy dishes. But it's also this heat component that is beneficial to pain relief.

When you ingest it, capsaicin works in the body like one of your neurotransmitters, or brain chemicals. It does this by binding with the vanilloid receptor 1 (VR1).

Why does it relieve pain? Well, when a heat increase is felt in the body, VR1 changes its shape and signals nerve cells to feel heat. The brain is actually "fooled" by capsaicin, however.

When you take capsaicin when you have pain, the brain thinks the heat signal from the capsaicin is actually an increased pain signal.

Capsaicin tricks the brain into reducing the pain (heat) signal by depleting the nerves of "substance P." And when substance P is depleted, the nerves can no longer send a pain signal to the brain.

There have been many clinical trials on the topical and ingested use of capsaicin for pain relief. In one double-blind clinical study, 70 patients with osteoarthritis (OA) and 31 with rheumatoid arthritis (RA) received capsaicin cream or placebo for a month for treatment of arthritic knee pain. The RA subjects experienced a 57% pain reduction, and the OA subjects had their pain reduced by 33%.

As the study paper concludes: *"According to the global evaluations, 80% of the capsaicin-treated patients experienced a reduction in pain after two weeks of treatment. It is concluded that capsaicin cream is a safe and effective treatment for arthritis."*

Another study on capsaicin for chronic neck pain found that applying topical capsaicin cream to the affected area four times daily for five weeks showed pain relief by deleting the sensory C-fibers of substance P.

There are hundreds more.

DELICIOUS PAIN RELIEF

Known the world over as a root for reducing stomach upset, nausea and motion sickness, not to mention making vegetables and chicken taste really good, ginger is effective in reducing inflammation, rheumatism and many kinds of pain.

In one study on the effects of ginger on rheumatism and musculoskeletal disorders, 56 patients were given powdered ginger. Of these, 28 had rheumatoid arthritis (RA), 19 had osteoarthritis (OA) and 10 had muscular discomfort. Over a period of three months to 2.5 years, an impressive 100% of participants with muscular discomfort experienced pain relief. What's more, 75% of arthritic participants experienced relief in pain and swelling. No adverse side effects were reported.

In another randomized, controlled study, women with painful menses were randomly assigned into two groups; one receiving ginger and the other placebo. Each received 500 mg capsules of ginger root powder (or placebo) three times daily. The researchers found, *"significant differences in the severity of pain between ginger and placebo groups."* And, *"treatment of primary (pain) in students with ginger for five days had a statistically significant effect on relieving intensity and duration of pain."*

Traditional cultures from around the world discovered through thousands of years of real world experience that food is medicine. Specifically, they found that thermogenic (heat inducing) spices like chili, turmeric and ginger (among others) are excellent at reducing inflammation and pain.

Including more of these spices in our meals, in their whole food states or in powdered spice incarnation, can do much to reduce chronic inflammation and pain. And eating tasty food with a bit of a kick has the added benefit of zero side effects, unlike taxing the body with too many anti-inflammatory pain meds.

TRY DMSO AND WIPE OUT PAIN AND INFLAMMATION

There comes a time when you just need to forget the approval of the Food and Drug Administration (FDA) and use a product that has been proven effective. Many effective treatments are available that lack sanctioning or approval for various reasons, including politics and bias. In this category, a product known as DMSO (dimethyl sulfoxide) is a useful substance that has a long history of being ignored, or even blackballed, yet has helped millions of people in pain.

ODD BEGINNINGS

DMSO has strong anti-inflammatory and analgesic properties. Originally a commercial solvent used in the wood industry in the early 1950s, DMSO was first applied in the medical field as a preservative for transporting organs during the 1960s. Stanley Jacob, MD, a former head of the organ transplant program at Oregon Health Sciences University in Portland, OR, started looking into its potential as a healing agent when he saw how fast and how deeply it penetrated the skin.

Since the '60s, more than 40,000 articles concerning DMSO have appeared in scientific journals. They show DMSO to have versatile properties and numerous health benefits. In fact, according to Terry Bristol, president of the Institute for Science, Engineering and Public Policy in Portland, DMSO was the first nonsteroidal antiinflammatory (NSAID) discovered after aspirin. He believes it is this product that spurred research into the development of other NSAIDs.

TOO GOOD FOR THE FDA?

As a result of its early heralding of being a "wonder" product, many companies tried to patent DMSO. However, the FDA rejected approval across the board, mainly because it has a wide range of attributes, not merely one (as drugs need for approval). In other words, a drug needs to be effective for a single illness, focusing on the symptoms and not the causes of health problems. This represents a perverse reversal of the perspective of traditional healing systems.

DMSO, however, violates the FDA's narrow requirement with its ability to help numerous health issues, including pain, inflammation, sprains, arthritis, stroke, clots, central nervous system trauma, minor cuts and burns (it speeds healing) as well as protection against cancerous cells. Yet, in the United States, DMSO has FDA approval only for use as a preservative of organs for transplant and for interstitial cystitis (a bladder disease).

QUICK BENEFITS

I love DMSO and use it as often as needed. Among the topical analgesics and anti-inflammatory products out there, it is among the safest and most effective. In fact, it stands perhaps alone in its ability to be administered topically, orally and intravenously.

When applied topically, it absorbs quickly into the skin and reaches deeper tissues and membranes. It has been found to be a great carrier of other substances, and it aids in their absorption. I sometimes use other topical pain/inflammation creams mixed with DMSO gel to help reduce pain and inflammation. When antifungals, cortisone and penicillin are mixed with a DMSO solution of between 70% and 90%, you get quicker and deeper penetration of the tissues. I use the 70% solution for regular pain, sprains, inflammation from exercise or daily strain. When there is particular pain or stiffness or inflammation, I use the 90% solution.

HOW AND WHY IT WORKS

DMSO has antioxidant properties. As such, it neutralizes free radicals around an injured site. It also stabilizes and stops leakage from damaged cell membranes. This combination effectively reduces inflammation. What's more, according to lab studies, DMSO reduces pain by blocking peripheral nerve C fibers.

It is thought that DMSO works because it is rich in sulfur. This element is among the most abundant in the body and plays a role in the formation of muscle, skin, hair and nails. Sulfur is also one of the building blocks of collagen, the connective tissue that makes up cartilage. Studies indicate that cartilage afflicted with degenerative arthritis contains low levels of sulfur. As such, DMSO is often used for those suffering arthritis and joint pain, though it is equally effective for muscle pain and spasms.

FORGET ABOUT FDA APPROVAL HERE

The way DMSO is viewed by the FDA is, to me, perverse. I subscribe to the traditional Chinese medicine (TCM) philosophy that a medicine (in the TCM case, herbal medicine) is considered "low" if it works on only one or two health issues. The TCM concept holds that many health issues arise from the same or similar root causes, so a remedy must treat the "root" (the cause) and not just the "branches" (the symptoms). Therefore, a remedy is considered "high" when it effectively treats multiple health concerns concurrently; this means it is correcting the root imbalance causing the symptoms. The FDA, with its single-use philosophy, misses the boat and will never approve safer and more powerful substances, like DMSO. And when it sanctions trials on Chinese herbals, it isolates individual compounds to then make them suitable for pharmaceutical (single-use) drugs. What a pity.

DMSO is available online. I get mine from Amazon. If you are suffering pain, inflammation, arthritis or other related ailments, give it a try. Do more research if you like; I list a number of articles at the end of the chapter for your reference. Remember, DMSO is safe and it works.

MAGNIFICENT MAGNESIUM

As a nation, Americans are woefully deficient in magnesium, a mineral vital for protection against soreness and pain. The tragedy is that getting enough magnesium is a simple matter, but it makes a world of difference for your health.

Research shows that only 25% of those living in the West consume sufficient levels of magnesium. That means the large majority, 75%, are deficient in this mineral. Why does this matter? Magnesium – along with calcium, iron, phosphorous, potassium and zinc – is a crucial macromineral necessary for optimal health. This means that we – along with much of the rest of the animal kingdom – need at least 100 mg per day to remain healthy. With the research showing that three out of four Westerners are deficient in magnesium, it's no wonder we are among the world's sickest people.

ABUNDANT SUBSTANCE

Magnesium is among the most abundant elements in the human body, where its ions are essential to living cells. It is a cofactor in the manipulation of compounds like adenosine triphosphate (ATP), the "universal energy molecule"), deoxyribonucleic acid (DNA) and ribonucleic acid (RNA), which are essential to human physiology. In fact, magnesium ions are necessary for hundreds of enzymes to function properly and help normalize hyperactive nerve function and vasoconstriction (spasm of blood vessels). It is easy to see how so much pain, illness and disease can be caused by magnesium deficiency.

According to Cornell University's Lawrence Resnicj, MD, *"A link between magnesium, diabetes and hypertension seems established beyond a reasonable doubt."*

Consider how magnesium influences these pain problems:

Muscle Spasm and Pain: More than 25% of the body's magnesium content is concentrated in the muscles. It helps deliver the correct amount of oxygen to the muscles to help them contract and relax, and it aids in the transmission of nerve impulses to them.

Fatigue: Magnesium helps convert carbohydrates we consume into usable energy. A deficiency of magnesium, then, can lead to extreme tiredness.

Migraines: Numerous studies show a direct link between those who suffer migraine headaches and low levels of magnesium. In their book, *What Your Doctor May Not Tell You About Migraines*, Alexander Mauskop and Barry Fox reported: *"A group of 3,000 patients given 200 mg of magnesium daily had an 80% reduction in their migraine symptoms."*

TYPES OF MAGNESIUM

The hundreds of essential functions within the human body requiring magnesium leave little doubt that maintaining adequate levels of magnesium is crucial to overall health and wellness. There are many ways to increase your magnesium intake, such as food and supplementation.

Natural food sources of magnesium include:

- Fruits: Oranges, bananas and cantaloupe
- Vegetables: Spinach, broccoli, zucchini, lima beans, cauliflower, artichokes and carrots
- Legumes: Pinto beans, lentils, chickpeas
- Nuts and seeds
- Potatoes

Supplemental sources of magnesium include:

- Magnesium Gluconate and Oxide: Often taken long-term to help maintain overall magnesium levels in the body.
- Magnesium Lactate: Sometimes used to treat indigestion and heartburn, and often used to correct magnesium deficiency.

- Magnesium Citrate: Often used to treat constipation.
- Magnesium Hydroxide: Often used as a laxative and an antacid.

CHECKING ON MAGNESIUM

It is important to speak to your physician or healthcare provider to have your magnesium levels checked. If you are suffering one or more of the common ailments associated with magnesium deficiency, it may be somewhat easy for you to overcome them. A diet high in magnesium-rich foods is the best place to start. If supplementation is needed or wanted, consult with your healthcare provider or knowledgeable expert at a health food store to determine which type of magnesium supplementation is best suited to your needs. I take 400 mg of chelated magnesium daily.

USE CHINESE TOPICAL TREATMENTS FOR PAIN RELIEF

When searching for relief from pain, inflammation, swelling and stiffness, many people reach for a topical cream, gel or ointment. These products fill the shelves of drugstores and supermarkets. Though the Eastern and Western versions of these products have some different ingredients, they serve the same purpose: instant relief from pain and stiffness.

Topical pain products are used mostly for short-term relief; as soon as their active ingredients have metabolized in the body, they just about stop killing the pain. For effectiveness over the long term, they should be applied three times a day, and be part of an overall program for arthritis relief. On their own, these products can provide almost instant relief on some level to one or more symptoms and can be used to help you get through your day or night.

How Topical Products Work

There are several key ways in which the various topical products help reduce pain, swelling, inflammation and stiffness. Many of the products are known as counterirritants; they irritate your skin in a way that shifts your mind and nervous system off the pain issue. In other words, ingredients like menthol, wintergreen oil and eucalyptus are used to counter the symptomatic irritant by creating a new irritant, like redness or sensations of cold or warmth on the skin.

This process is also known as "gate control" or "gating." It gates off or blocks the receptors in the skin from sending pain signals to the brain, instead stimulating them to send a heating or cooling signal. This "tricks" the mind into focusing on the new irritant. In turn, that convinces the nervous system that the area is hot (drawing increased circulation) or cold (metabolically warming the area). Those actions improve the bothersome symptoms.

Many of the topical products contain salicylates, a class of chemicals that acts in a way similar to NSAIDs (nonsteroidal anti- inflammatory drugs). These chemicals appear naturally in mint, menthol and peppermint, for example, and in aspirin. They work by inhibiting the synthesis of prostaglandin, the naturally occurring and chemically related fatty acids that aid in blood pressure and body temperature regulation and that control inflammation and vascular permeability.

A Look at the Common Ingredients

Many of the most popular pain-relieving creams and gels share common ingredients like wintergreen, camphor, menthol, capsaicin and salicylate. Here is a brief overview of each component.

Wintergreen: The oil made from wintergreen leaf is often applied locally at the site of pain for treatment of arthritis, rheumatism, lower back pain, sciatica, headache and menstrual cramps. It is also used for pain, swelling, fever and nausea. In high concentrations, wintergreen acts as a counterirritant. Once wintergreen is absorbed into the skin and metabolized by the body, it changes into a salicylate and then acts like an NSAID. If you have allergies to aspirin or salicylates, do not use products containing wintergreen oil. If not, give them a try.

Menthol: An organic compound derived from the mentha (mint, peppermint) family of plants, menthol is one of nature's best analgesics, for three reasons:

- When menthol is included in a delivery agent, like topical creams, molecules called ligands attach themselves to receptors in your cells, triggering a change.
- Menthol triggers vasodilation or the expanding of blood vessels.

This expansion allows extra blood flow to the area.

- Menthol is an antipyretic, meaning it has a natural cooling effect that fools the nervous system into thinking the body is cold. This leads the nerves to send back a signal that relieves the heat of inflammation.

Camphor Oil: Extracted from two types of camphor trees, this is a stimulant that calms nerve pain, reduces inflammation and is used as an anesthetic, disinfectant and sedative. While camphor has a cooling effect on the area on which it is applied, it stimulates blood flow, helps metabolism and causes the sweating of fluids, especially in and around the joints, to reduce swelling. Its cooling nature makes it a great anti-inflammatory agent. It is very useful at reducing pain through its temporary numbing of the sensory nerves and its vasoconstriction (blood vessel contraction). Those actions take pressure off swelling around nerves. Camphor oil is a toxic substance that can be fatal if ingested in doses as little as 2 grams. External use only!

Capsaicin: The compound that gives the chili its heat and pungency and is the aspect that helps with pain symptoms. While the hot feeling conveyed by capsaicin may feel harsh at first, it does lessen with time. It is a counterirritant that produces a hot, burning sensation on the skin where applied, tricking the brain into thinking the area is hot and attracting blood flow that helps with stiffness, pain and hyperactive nerve firing. Capsaicin also works by diminishing the chemical in the body known as substance P, which is involved in transmitting pain signals to the brain.

Going Beyond Common Brands and Ingredients

Reaching for brands like BENGAY® and IcyHot® is OK, if that is all you have available. However, I'd like to introduce you to a few topical products from traditional Chinese medicine (TCM).

White Flower Analgesic Balm: An analgesic balm that works as a natural pain reliever for aching joints, headaches, sprains and backache. It contains wintergreen, menthol and camphor and also combines the essential oils derived from lavender, eucalyptus and peppermint. It is a potent aromatherapy agent that has a soothing and calming effect on the nerves and emotions.

Red Flower Oil: This oil is good for treating acute and chronic joint pain, muscle aches, sprains and bruising. In addition to wintergreen and camphor, red flower oil blends several essential oils. These include clove, cinnamon and turpentine (alpha pinene).

Po Sum On Oil: A warming liniment with pain-relieving and anti-inflammatory effects. It is uniquely made from menthol plus the essential oils of peppermint, tea, dragon blood resin, cinnamon, scute and licorice. Peppermint oil is both an analgesic (pain reliever) and antispasmodic (muscle relaxer). Dragon blood is a resin that aids in blood circulation and tissue regeneration. Cinnamon oil is a stimulant that aids blood circulation and reduces pain. Scute and licorice both help alleviate skin inflammation.

Wong Lop Kong Medicated Oil: Wong Lop Kong is one of my favorite medicated oils from Asia because it truly employs both essential oils and traditional Chinese herbal therapy. It contains camphor, safflower, peppermint, tea oil, frankincense gum resin and myrrh. Wong Lop Kong also contains dragon's blood resin, dang gui (angelica), salvia root (danshen) and ligusticum (chuanxiong), making this topical product great for muscle and joint pain, rheumatism, bruises, blood clots and sprains.

All of these products are available in Chinatowns and Asian markets. If you don't live near one, you can simple do an online search and grab one online.

Please read the labels of any of the products you are going to use prior to applying to your body. Many are harmful if applied to open wounds and scratches, if they touch the eyes or are accidentally ingested. Aside from that, applying to the painful area three times a day should offer enough relief to make a difference.

DO YOU HAVE PEPPERMINT OIL IN YOUR MEDICINE CABINET?

The best medicines are the ones that have many uses and applications. In Asian medicine, if an herb has only one or two applications, it is considered insignificant. Because ailments, diseases and pain do not happen in a vacuum, it is important that any treatment do more than one thing.

Essential oils do just that. Peppermint oil, in particular, is broadly effective at treating and easing a number of issues related to health and wellness.

Peppermint oil is among the so-called "essential oils" used in naturopathic medicine and various healing traditions. The oils of the peppermint plant (including leaves, stems, roots) are distilled into a concentrated liquid, or "oil." This oil is said to contain the "essence" of the plant and is quite strong; as such, it is often mixed with a carrier oil (like almond, grapeseed or jojoba) to help dilute it before use. Some people have a red or rash-like response in they have sensitive skin.

WHY PEPPERMINT?

You can apply peppermint essential oil directly to the skin, inhale it via steam or aromatherapy device, consume it in foods and beverages, or add it to enemas to effect a symptomatic relief for such things as stomach upset, respiratory issues, muscle pain and more.

It works in part because the peppermint plant contains menthol, which is a local anesthetic. When applied topically, the area feels warm and blood is drawn to it as a method to relieve pain, tightness and tension.

It's no wonder menthol and peppermint are ingredients in so many topical analgesic gels and creams. In addition, peppermint oil is said to have anti-inflammatory, antispasmodic, antibacterial and antiviral properties.

While peppermint essential oil has been linked to dozens of health benefits, including use in cancer treatment and regrowth of hair; we'll take a look here at its pain relief properties:

FIGHT HEADACHES AND MIGRAINES

Headaches and migraines are horrible because they are not only painful but are centered in your head, where you do your thinking, making it hard to work. When mixed with a carrier oil, a few drops of peppermint oil can help relieve the symptoms of a headache, or prevent them at first sign in some cases. Simply rub a few drops onto your temples, along your forehead and over your sinuses for soothing relief. Remember, there are anti-inflammatory and analgesic properties at work as well as heat to draw fresh blood and oxygen to the areas. For tension type headaches, massage a few drops into the neck and shoulders and under the occiput (base of the skull resting above the spine).

EASE MUSCLE STRAIN

Peppermint oil's natural analgesic, antispasmodic and anti-inflammatory properties again come to the fore in their use to relax and relieve muscle strain, spasm and tightness caused by such things as stress, poor posture or too much physical exertion. Simply rub peppermint oil onto the skin above the affected muscle(s) and massage the area. The menthol will bring fresh blood into the muscles and the other properties just mentioned will prevent or reduce spams, trigger point and reduce pain.

PERFECT STRESS RELIEF

Aromatherapy is a common and much-trusted remedy for psychological stress. Adding peppermint oil drops to a warm bath, rubbing a few drops on your wrists or diffusing the oil with an aromatherapy device are great ways to inhale and relax away the tension of the day. People who use peppermint oil as aromatherapy daily report less stress, tension and anxiety, which can all help aid digestion, sleep and mental health.

POTENTIAL SIDE EFFECTS

Although peppermint oil has many wonderful uses and benefits, like anything else it does have a few side effects. The most common is irritation of the skin when applied directly without a carrier oil to reduce concentration. Another to be aware of is consuming peppermint oil supplements if you have an issue with producing enough hydrochloric acid in the stomach. The oil can irritate the stomach in this case. And do not ingest peppermint oil when you have diarrhea for it may cause anal burning. Aside from this, peppermint oil's broad spectrum of uses makes it a keeper in my book.

REFERENCES:

The anti-cancer secret from India.

Turmeric: Nature's Powerful Anti-Inflammatory Root.

Treatment of arthritis with topical capsaicin: a double-blind trial.
Topical capsaicin for chronic neck pain. A pilot study.

The influence of local capsaicin treatment on small nerve fibre function and neurovascular control in symptomatic diabetic neuropathy.

Effect of Zingiber officin.zomes (ginger) on pain relief in primary dysmenorrhea: a placebo randomized trial.

Ginger (Zingiber officinale) in rheumatism and musculoskeletal disorders. Kolb KH, Jaenicke G, Krame, M, Schulze PE. Absorption, distribution, and elimination of labeled dimethyl sulfoxide in man and animals. Ann NY Acad Sci. 141:85-95, 1967.

Evans MS, Reid KH, Sharp JB. Dimethyl sulfoxide (DMSO) blocks conduction in peripheral nerve C fibers: A possible mechanism of analgesia.

Neurosci Lett. 150:145-148, 1993.

Demos CH, Beckloff G, Donin MN, Oliver PM. Dimethyl sulfoxide in musculoskeletal disorders. Ann NY Acad Sci. 141:517-523, 1967.

Lockie LM, Norcross B. A clinical study on the effects of dimethyl sulfoxide in 103 patients with acute and chronic musculoskeletal injures and inflammation. Ann NY Acad Sci. 141:599-602, 1967.

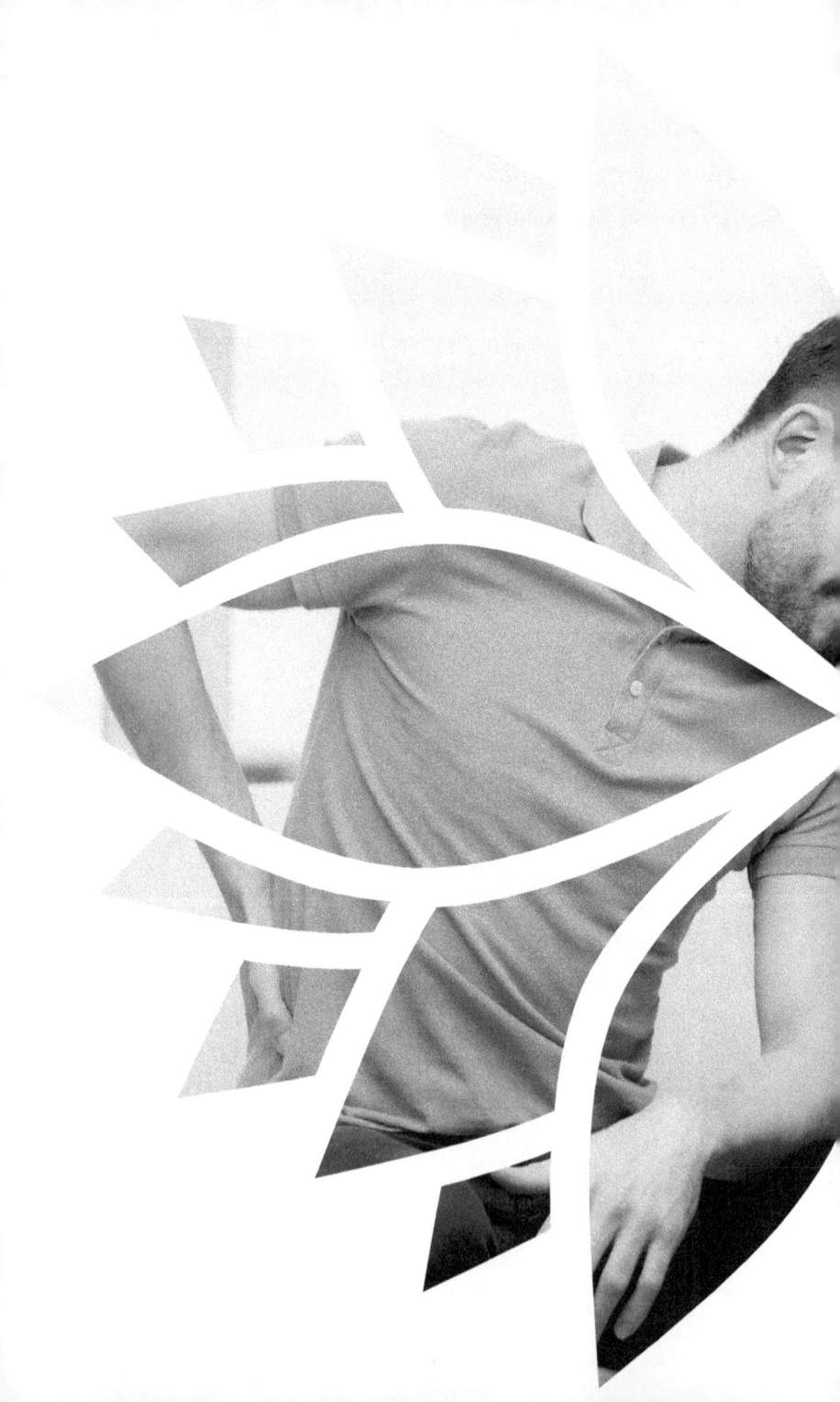

CHAPTER 8

DEALING WITH LOW BACK PAIN, THE WORLD'S NO. 1 HEALTH PROBLEM

*I*n 2013, *The Lancet* published the results of the largest ever systematic effort that was carried out to describe just how and where in the world major diseases, injuries and health risk factors were most prevalent. This study, "The Global Burden of Disease Study 2010," is divided into seven sections, each on a specific disease and the effects on the world population. It included heart disease, cancer, injuries and other conditions.

The analysis showed that although the human race has increased its life expectancy by about 10 years since the 1970s, today men and women spend more years suffering injury, pain and illness than ever before. In other words, that additional decade of life expectancy created for us by modern science, technology and medicine has not produced a better quality of life – especially not during the final decade of life.

LONGER LIFE IS NO CAKE WALK

The Annals of the Rheumatic Diseases published a review and analysis of the Global Burden data in an effort to estimate the total global burden of low back pain. What they found: Worldwide, out of the nearly 300 conditions studied, low back pain (LBP) is the leading cause of disability and ranks as sixth in terms of overall disability burden. The study conclusion: *"LBP causes more global disability than any other condition. With the aging (sic) population, there is an urgent need for further research to better understand LBP across different settings."*

The most serious health problem: Not famine. Not AIDS. Not heart disease… but low back pain.

LOW BACK PAIN IS THE LEADING CULPRIT

The same research group that carried out this research published additional findings in the journal Arthritis & Rheumatism where they set out to examine the details of LBP, including prevalence period, case definition and other variables.

They conducted a systematic review of the global prevalence of low back pain that included general population studies published between 1980 and 2009. A total of 165 studies from 54 countries were analyzed. Of these, 64% had been published since the last comparable review.

This additional review indicated that LBP is indeed a massive problem worldwide. Moreover, women between the ages of 40 and 80 are most at risk. In other words, this demographic group suffered the greatest prevalence of injury and disability due to low back pain.

THE LOW BACK PAIN PUZZLE

In these three pieces of research, it seems those conducting the studies were successful in uncovering a major problem, yet were unable to pinpoint a unifying cause, a global cause or a solution. They know that all over the world a remarkably large number of people suffer with low back pain and are disabled by it, but they cannot say why or suggest what to do.

The medical community is puzzled by this.

MY THOUGHTS

There are many causes for low back pain. These include:

Soft Tissue Damage: Causes include twisting too hard, bending over for too long, lifting something overly heavy and sleeping in an odd position. These actions can cause micro tears to the tendons and ligaments or cause the muscles of the lower back to seize up, stiffen and either compress or bind nerves, reducing the flow of blood. They may also cause inflammation. Any of these can lead to disabling pain and discomfort.

Skeletal Trauma: Causes include injury to the low back from such things as a hard fall, auto accident and other physically damaging actions. Can also be linked to infections, viruses and bacteria that result in spinal degeneration, deterioration of the spinal cord and erosion of the spinal discs. These can all lead to various kinds of pain and disability.

Psychological Distress: Stress, anxiety, fear and a traumatic emotional event can all set in motion a nervous system response that restricts blood and oxygen flow and distribution in addition to causing inflammation and the release of bio-chemicals that adversely affect health.

Dietary Issues: A diet low in natural calcium, magnesium, potassium and other essential nutrients can lead to poor development of the spine and other parts of the body. The brain controls the nervous system; the skeleton holds the body and allows for mobility and action via the joints; the muscles, ligaments and tendons move the limbs to do work. When the body is deficient in essential nutrients like glucose, potassium, magnesium, sodium, calcium, iron, zinc, selenium, the B vitamins and so on, it will not be in optimal functioning shape. Malnutrition can lead to a weak body and a weak low back that puts you at increased risk for disabling low back pain from soft-tissue damage and skeletal trauma. Nutritional deficiencies also play a role in essential hormonal balances that can lead to depression, anxiety and other psychologically distressing states that, themselves, lead to low back pain.

SIMPLE SOLUTIONS TO A HUGE PROBLEM

Please excuse me if I attempt to oversimplify this massive global problem. But, in general, I have found that when a patient with a health problem describes his problem to a healthcare provider, he frames it in a way he believes is useful to the provider. He doesn't describe the complete situation that has led to the problem.

For example, when a patient with low back pain describes the pain to a primary care physician, he discusses the physical pain and physical discomfort. Omitted are the psychological factors he might discuss with a psychotherapist, things like the fact that the pain starts after an argument with his spouse.

Patients are also reluctant to bring up subjects they think will reflect poorly on their character.

I believe that if people worldwide could understand that there are many causes of low back pain, and that each cause requires a different cure – sometimes anti-inflammatories, sometimes massage, sometimes psychological therapy, sometimes dietary changes – then each person could play a stronger role in preventing and treating this condition.

This takes some insight on the part of the individual. When dealing with back pain, you are to be mindful of your life's circumstances and your activities, both physical and emotional. That allows you to focus on the moment when the pain starts and grasp more fully why it occurs.

From this small amount of personal insight and assessment, you experiment to see which therapy helps relieve your pain. Use some trial and error. Low back pain is (in most cases) not disease-related. Therefore, it is within our grasp as individuals to prevent it and relieve the planet of this epidemic.

HOW TO STOP BACK PAIN AND SAVE YOUR SPINE FROM SWAYBACK

When spinal health is compromised by muscle imbalances and postural changes, low back pain and limited range of motion can keep you from doing what you love.

Maintaining your natural s-curve is essential to proper muscle balance and range of motion as you age – which means mobility and independence… and no back pain.

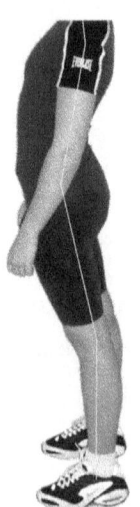

One common problem that occurs is known as swayback posture. Those who develop swayback often experience muscle tightness, trigger points, tears, inflammation, pain and limited mobility in the lower back, legs and hips. This can mean a decreased quality of life because of an inability to carry out daily activities or sports and recreation without great effort or discomfort.

LOWER BODY HYPEREXTENSION

Swayback posture is the result of postural changes in the pelvis and thighs which causes hyperextension of the knees and hips.

Picture someone standing with knees locked back and pelvis protruding forward. This causes a sway in the back and thus alters posture overall, and physical function. Swayback is easy to see in someone's posture by the way they stand. No matter their weight or fitness level, their belly will protrude forward because of a forward pelvic tilt. And their shoulders will rest backward of the hips and you'll also see a forward head posture.

It is not uncommon for people to misdiagnose hyperlordosis with swayback. But here is a telltale difference: Lordosis finds the lumbar (lower) spine in a concave position while with swayback the lumbar spine is actually flattened with the concave curvature in the thoracic (mid) spine. Neither diagnosis is good, but differentiation is the key to correcting the swayback posture.

DANGERS OF SWAYBACK

Any kind of postural dysfunction is bad and each has its own way of affecting one's life. Among the dangers of uncorrected swayback is overuse of the hamstrings (muscle group on back of the thighs) by virtue of firing them to extend the hips rather than the gluteal (butt) muscles. This improper posture is bad for the joints and overtime causes wear-and-tear on the femur (thigh bone) and hip ball-and-socket joints. Aside from muscle spasms, trigger points in the hamstring and tendonitis, this can cause reduction of cartilage and eventually leads to osteoarthritis.

Functionally speaking, people who maintain this postural dysfunction develop tight hip flexors which can be painful while also reducing range of motion in step, stretch and bend, making it difficult to bend to tie shoes or pick something up off the floor, or walk long distances up slopes or stairs.

HIGH HEELS, HIGH RISK

Like most postural dysfunctions, and the pain and restrictions associated with them, swayback is preventable and reversible because it is caused by our own postural choices. The problem is that many of us don't know we are causing it.

To begin, those who walk in high heels are practically forcing the swayback postures on themselves. The heels change the ankle position, move the center of gravity, and cause swayback posture. Yes, this is temporary but those who wear high heels frequently may end up with a muscle memory that creates a chronic swayback posture.

Stomach sleeping is also a cause of swayback because the lower back is not supported during this sleep position. While stomach sleeping, the abdomen sinks into the mattress, which pulls on the lower back, causing the body to hold a swayback posture for hours on end. Very bad. It is best to sleep on your side or your back if you have this issue.

CORRECTING SWAYBACK POSTURE

While swayback posture can lead to chronic pain, limited range of motion and decreased quality of life, the good news is that it can be reversed and the problems avoided. A few simple exercises done at least once, preferably three times per day is great, and will do much to correct the muscle imbalances leading to this postural dysfunction.

1) Stretch and Strengthen the Hip Flexors – The basic method is to both stretch and strengthen the shortened hip flexors. The stretch to get you started is to take a deep and long lunge forward, then lower your back knee toward the floor.

You can strengthen the flexors by doing the "mountain climbing" drill on the floor. From a push up position, you are like running in place.

2) Strengthen the Glutes – Remember, glutes are your butt muscles and these can be strengthened in several ways. First lie on your back with knees bent, feet flat on floor and arms at your sides for balance. Now do a bridge movement by slowly raising your hips up off the floor and then slowly lowering them for as many as makes you tired. You should feel the tension and burn in the butt!

Next are clams, which find you on your side, legs bent and parallel to one another. Slowly open and close the top leg until tired and then turn over and repeat on the other leg.

3) Tighten the Abs – Shortening the external obliques or stomach muscles will do much to hold the core in place and prevent swaying. You want to strengthen in two ways. Windshield wipers are a good place to start. Lie on your back with arms extended out to their respective sides for balance. Raise both legs up straight and rotate them from side to side together, like windshield wipers. Try to do 10 or as many as you can and improve from there.

Next are side bends with dumbbells. Stand up straight while holding a hand weight (dumbbell) in one hand; the other hand is placed behind the back of your head. Now bend toward the floor, sideways, in the direction of the hand holding the weight, and then raise back to vertical position. Again, 10 reps should do it, then switch hands and do the other side.

Like so many common wellness issues swayback posture is caused, and can be reversed, by our choices and actions. Knowledge is power, so first knowing there is an issue and how it is caused will give you the information to stop doing the things that create the postural dysfunction. Second, is the knowledge of basic things that you can do to correct the muscle imbalances that create the issue. Now that you know, have fun making positive changes to your body that will positively affect your wellbeing and help you lose the back pain.

POWER THROUGH WORK OR PLAY WITH NO BACK PAIN

If you sit in an office, car or truck most of the day, low back pain may afflict you unmercifully. But instead of reaching for anti-inflammatory and analgesic pills as a first response, you can relieve the symptoms of low back and hip pain naturally.

Sitting shortens muscles in the low back, hips and legs and cuts off your circulation. You can find pain relief in exercise, stretching, yoga and massage. And prevention is always more effective than reacting to active pain: Stretch the muscle groups that tend to tighten (shorten) as a result of sitting for extended periods every day to stop the discomfort before it starts.

STOPPING THE PAIN

If you're too busy or broke to visit a masseuse or to attend a yoga class, you can design your own pain-relief program. In just a few minutes per day in your office using only your chair, you can stretch (elongate) those tight muscles and return them to their normal resting, comfortable length and bring fresh blood, oxygen and nutrients into their tissues. This reduces pain, increases range of motion and reduces or prevents low back pain caused from sitting too long.

The muscles most responsible for creating low back pain are hip flexors, glutes, hamstrings, adductors and quadriceps.

The tensor fasciae latae (TFL) is responsible for flexing, abducting (moving away from the body's midline) and medially rotating the hip joints. The gluteus medius and minimus both abduct and medially rotate the hip joints. When the tensor fasciae latae, gluteus medius and gluteus minimus are tight, they can cause imbalances in the pelvis, which can lead to hip, low back and outer knee pain. The gluteus maximus laterally rotates the hips and also abducts the thigh when the hip is flexed. When tight, the gluteus maximus can constrict the sciatic nerve, causing pain in the hip and down the back of the leg.

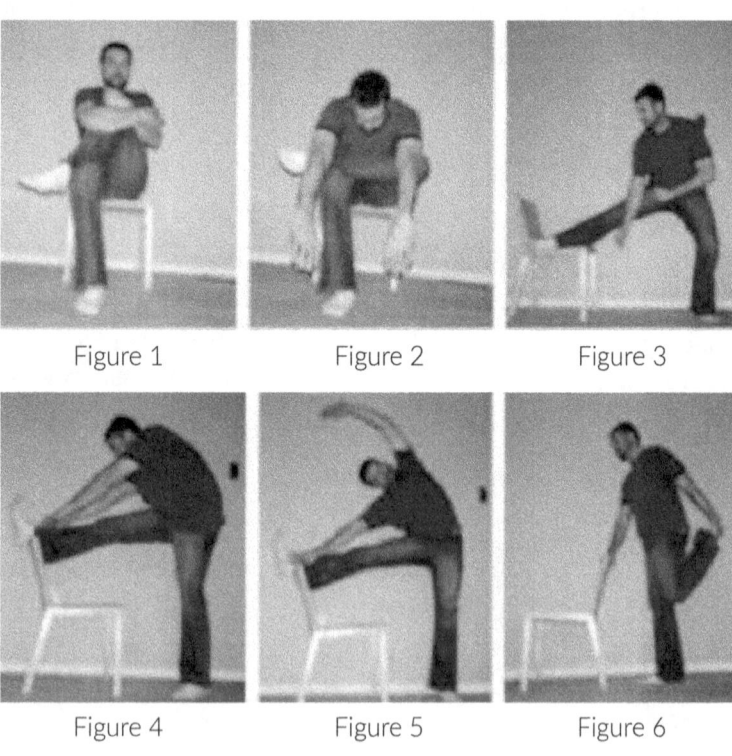

Figure 1　　　　Figure 2　　　　Figure 3

Figure 4　　　　Figure 5　　　　Figure 6

STRETCHES AT WORK

To stretch this series of muscles while seated at work, simply cross the ankle of one foot over the knee of the opposite leg and pull your knee toward your chest. Hold for 30 seconds and slowly release. Do this three times, then repeat on the opposite side. (Fig. 1)

Like the gluteus maximus, the piriformis laterally rotates the hips and abducts the thigh when the hips are flexed. Also, when tight, the piriformis may compress the sciatic nerve and cause pain in the hips, buttocks and down the back of the leg.

To stretch the piriformis while seated at work, simply cross the ankle of one foot over the knee of the opposite leg and bend forward at the waist. Hold for 30 seconds and slowly release. Do this three times, and then repeat on the opposite side. (Fig. 2)

The adductors are a group of three muscles that include the adductor brevis, adductor longus and adductor magnus. All three of these adduct (move toward the body's midline) and laterally rotate the hips, while the longus and brevis also flex and extend the femur. When tight, the adductors can cause groin pulls and make it somewhat uncomfortable or painful to do activities like ride a horse or play soccer.

To stretch the adductors while at work, stand perpendicular to your chair and place the foot of the closest leg on the chair and bend the supporting leg a bit until a stretch along the inner leg is felt. Hold for 30 seconds and slowly release. Do this three times, then repeat on the opposite side. (Fig. 3)

Three muscles form the group called the hamstrings. These include the biceps femoris, semitendinosus and semimembranosus. These are responsible for flexing the knee, extending the hips and rotating the lower legs. When tight, the hamstrings can cause low back pain and knee pain, especially when walking or running.

To stretch the hamstrings while at work, stand facing your chair and raise one leg, placing the foot on the back of the chair, and bend forward with hands extended. Hold for 30 seconds and slowly release. Do this three times, then repeat on the opposite side. (Fig. 4)

You can also add to this by turning so you are perpendicular to the chair and then reaching sideways and over your head with the arm of the side of the body with the supporting leg (Fig. 5). This will also stretch the quadratus lumborum (QL), which laterally flexes the spinal column. When tight, the QL can restrict sideways bending and cause pain in the low back, hips and buttocks.

Four muscles combine to make up the quadriceps, including the rectus femoris, vastus lateralis, vastus medialis and vastus intermedius. The three vasti muscles extend the knees, and the rectus both extends the knees and flexes the hips. When tight, the quads can cause low back and knee pain.

To stretch the hamstrings while at work, stand facing the back of your chair and hold with one arm to stabilize your balance. Bend the knee of one leg and grab the ankle with the hand of the same-side arm. Hold for 30 seconds and slowly release. Do this three times, and then repeat on the opposite side. (Fig. 6)

Working in an office nowadays may have you sitting for almost your entire working day. Stretching in your office or at home is the most efficient way to relieve pain from sitting too long. These simple stretches can help relax these muscles, relieve acute low back, hip and knee pain, and prevent it from becoming chronic. And don't forget to stay hydrated by drinking plenty of water.

REFERENCES:

http://www.thelancet.com/themed/global-burden-of-disease

http://ard.bmj.com/content/early/2014/02/14/annrheumdis-2013 204428.short?g=w_ard_ahead_tab

http://onlinelibrary.wiley.com/doi/10.1002/art.34347/abstract

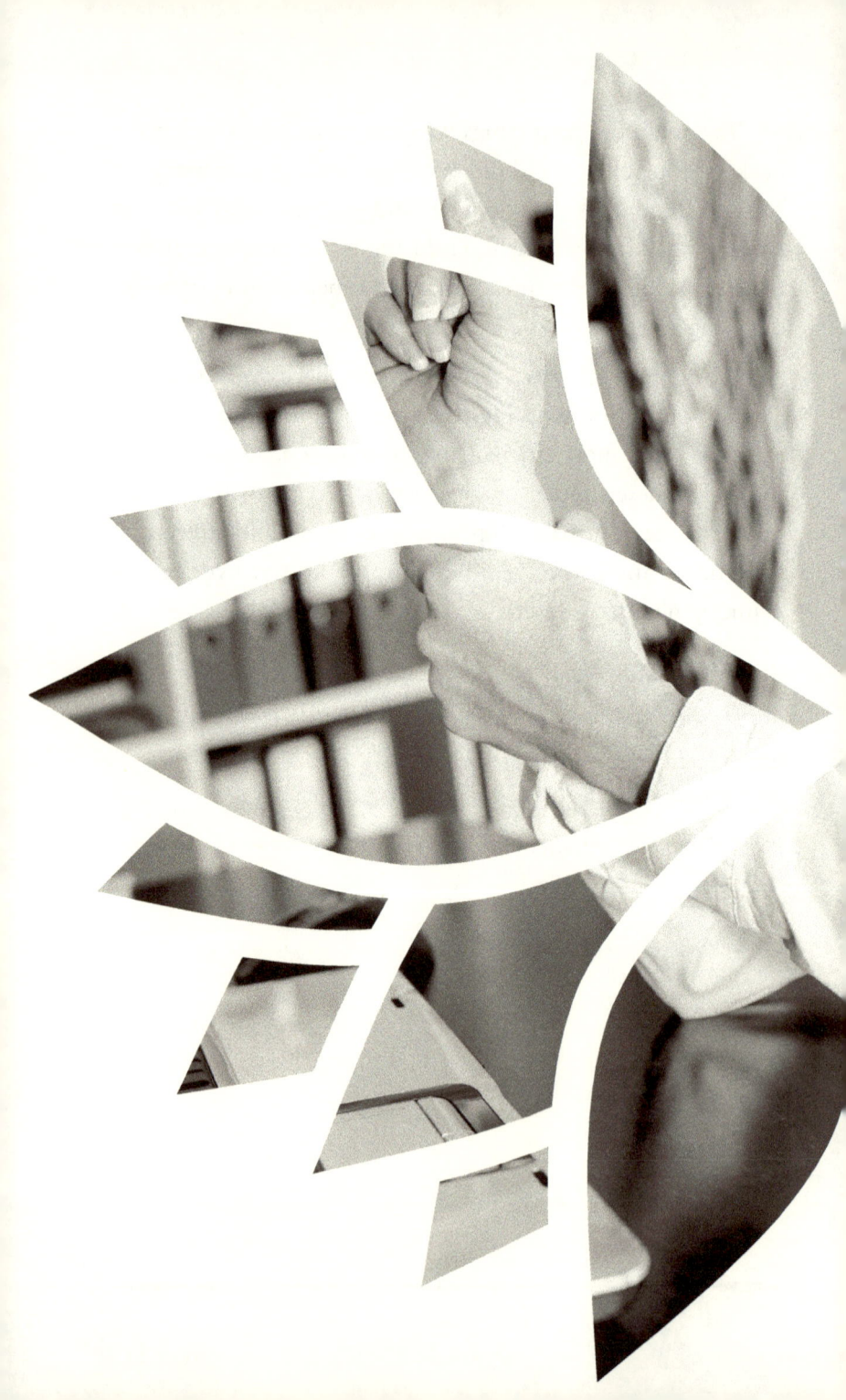

CHAPTER 9

JOINT PAIN GONE! EASY TRICKS TO RELIEVE KNEE, CARPAL TUNNEL, HAND AND WRIST PAIN

NATURAL APPROACHES FOR ALLEVIATING KNEE PAIN

Knee pain is among the most common types of pain for which people seek medical advice and treatment. Nonsteroidal anti-inflammatory drugs (NSAIDs), steroid injections and surgery seem to be more common than not. But they don't have to be. Naturally reducing symptoms and preventing further wear and tear can do much to prevent the problem from returning, and restoring quality of life.

THE KNEE JOINT

The knee joint is taken for granted to do what it needs to do to balance, bear weight, propel, raise and lower you. The knee is a hinge joint, which means it is meant to move back and forth from front to back, and not bend or twist or rotate side to side. Yet, this is what happens when playing sports or moving too quickly before ample warmup.

To help facilitate weight absorption and body movement the knee must rely on a bunch of muscles, tendons, ligaments and bones all working in tandem. When one piece of the puzzle is too tight, too weak, over developed or stiff – sprains, strains, dislocations and spurs can occur.

KNEE PAIN AND ARTHRITIS

When one seeks medical advice for knee pain in their 30s or older, they are often given a diagnosis of osteoarthritis. If you have been given an arthritis diagnosis, please don't let that word derail your efforts at natural relief and prevention. As we age, most people will get some form of arthritis or wear and tear on their joints. It's natural and normal, so don't be afraid of the diagnosis label. Read my advice on the "Top 10 Arthritis Mistakes" in chapter 11, or check out my book **Arthritis Reversed** for a comprehensive program. Among the most important components of any pain reduction program, is reduction of inflammation.

THE INFLAMMATION RESPONSE

Inflammation is a natural response your body has to stress, whether emotional or physical. The inflammation response helps protect the injured area and also to repair it. However, inflammation that does not resolve itself and becomes chronic is cause for concern, as it can cause serious health problems and disease. Chronic inflammation breaks your body's internal balance point, disrupts its ability to regulate the immune system and affects the functions of the central nervous system. As such, under the influence of chronic low-grade inflammation, you run a greater risk for pain, illness, disease and accelerated signs and symptoms of aging. The advice below will help you reduce inflammation, and thus pain, naturally.

PRICE-LESS FIRST LINE ADVICE

If you injure your knee or suddenly feel pain there, the acronym PRICE is a good reminder of what can help in the short run. It stands for Protect, Rest, Ice, Compress and Elevate. Here's the overview:

- Protecting the knee from additional trauma can be done by reducing or stropping activities that stress the joint too much, and wrapping the knee to keep it protected from fall or impact while recovering.
- Resting the knee allows it to begin repair while also preventing repetitive strain. But don't keep it immobile for too long or you may also develop frozen joint syndrome.

- Icing the knee will help reduce pain and inflammation in the short run, say 20 minutes at a time, several times that day.
- Compressing the knee also helps reduce swelling and pain by holding sustained pressure to promote circulation and holding the bones in alignment to prevent rub.
- Elevating the knee to above the heart will reduce swelling by allowing gravity to help circulate accumulated fluids around the knee.

APPLY SOME DMSO

As mentioned previously, DMSO is an old-timey product that athletes used to use for sprains and strains. I love it. Unlike other topical pain creams or ointments (which remain largely on skin surface), DMSO absorbs quickly into the skin and reaches deeper tissues and membranes.

It has been found to be a great carrier of other substances, and it aids in their absorption. I sometimes use other topical pain/inflammation creams mixed with DMSO gel to help reduce pain and inflammation.

Because DMSO has antioxidant properties it neutralizes free radicals around an injured site. It also stabilizes and stops leakage from damaged cell membranes and reduces pain by blocking peripheral nerve C fibers. DMSO is rich in sulfur, one of the building blocks of collagen, the connective tissue that makes up cartilage. As such, DMSO is often used for those suffering arthritis and joint pain, though it is equally effective for muscle pain and spasms.

FOUR WAYS TO KILL KNEE PAIN WITHOUT SURGERY

The effects of knee pain are many and often life-changing for the worse. This is why I offer natural solutions. Please consider putting these options to use before even thinking about orthoscopic or reconstructive knee surgery. They have proven to be largely unsuccessful, and useless, in studies and patient reports. Exhaust all other means before discussing surgery in a serious way, and with so many natural solutions available, relief should not be far away.

IMPROVING YOUR DIET

Diet is a contributor to inflammation and pain, and also can help reduce it. An anti-inflammatory and pain-reduction diet is easy, tastes great, is healthy and should include:

- **Green leafy vegetables** – collard greens, spinach, kale, Swiss chard, rainbow chard, turnip greens and mustard greens.
- **Fish, Fish oil, Seafood** – omega-3 fatty acids (in seafood or supplements), salmon, tuna, sardines, herring, trout and mussels.
- **Thermogenic spices** – garlic, ginger, turmeric, mustard, cayenne, onion and cloves.

Diet is a long-term plan for prevention of inflammation and reduction of pain because it takes a while for the foods to build up enough in the system to effect change. So start right away and continue your anti-inflammatory food lifestyle change!

SUPPORTING THE JOINT

Because there are so many things that intersect and cross the knee joint, keeping the upper and lower muscles in balance is essential to retain a strong structure, and reduce unnatural movement. When there are imbalances in the musculature of the calf, thigh and hamstring muscles, the knees can be pulled unnaturally to one side while being much weaker on the other. This occurs when ones quadriceps are over-developed but their hamstrings are weaker, or when their calves are too tight or too weak, and either create strain by pull or cannot match the larger thigh muscles in carrying a load or moving the body. Go to www.easyhealthoptions.com and click on "Exercise & Fitness" to search for an easy exercise to help balance the knee structures.

EXPLORING THE EMOTIONAL COMPONENT TO PAIN

Pain occurs for more reasons than just physical strain. If not, how does one explain the sudden knee pain or low back pain of a person who sits all day at work and at home, and does not engage in strenuous activities? The problem is that many people, and physicians, don't acknowledge or simply ignore the emotional, psychosomatic causes of pain. And yet, it is more prevalent than you'd think, and can be classified as Tension Myositis Syndrome (TMS).

TMS is a musculoskeletal neurological disorder created by the mind and emotions that changes one's physiology and causes pain and other symptoms. Essentially, it is believed that stress and repressed emotions like anger and anxiety are the root cause of chronic pain and a host of other disorders like tension headache, fibromyalgia, irritable bowel syndrome (IBS), constipation, arm pain, temporal mandibular joint dysfunction (TMJD) and tinnitus (ringing in the ears).

TMS case studies show that as the emotional components are dealt with successfully, the physical ailments that were heretofore intractable disappear almost instantly. The TMS diagnosis offers the potential to a powerful tool for relief of chronic pain.

IF NEEDED, LOSE SOME WEIGHT

Whether you are very overweight or just a little heavy, losing weight will decrease knee pain, improve knee joint function and reduce inflammation because it recused the load placed on the joint. Each pound of body fat equals about five pounds of load on the joints. So losing even a little weight will help immediately, and losing 10% of your body weight or more (when healthy enough to do so), can bring great results.

"HELP, I CAN'T TYPE!" OR HOW TO GET CARPAL TUNNEL RELIEF STARTING TODAY

Carpal tunnel syndrome (CTS) is a debilitating condition that can hamper your life. It hurts, period. The incessant pain, numbness and tingling are annoying and often overwhelming.

Moreover, carpal tunnel changes the way people work and do tasks with their hands. Gripping and holding become difficult and painful; typing or doing fine finger work (like electrics or sewing) can become nearly impossible. While surgery tends to provide the best relief, it often has unwanted side effects. I'd like to share another method of treatment, a do-it-yourself acupressure method that just may offer significant help.

THE NARROW CARPAL TUNNEL

The carpal tunnel is a narrow, rigid canal or passageway on the under (palm) side of the wrist. The area consists of bones, connective tissue, tendons and the median nerve. The carpal tunnel joins the forearm with the palm of the hand.

CARPAL TUNNEL SYNDROME

Carpal tunnel syndrome occurs when the medium nerve running through the carpal canal becomes irritated or compressed because of a narrowing of the canal area. Since this nerve is what sends the sensation signals to the palmar side of the hand, thumb and fingers (minus the pinky), compression leads to inflammation, pain, tingling and numbness. Other discomforts can include burning, itching, pain that radiates up the arm and weakness. Even when no visual swelling is apparent, sufferers feel like their hands are swollen, generally as a result of the numbness in the fingers.

CTS CAUSES

There are a number of things that can cause or put you at risk for developing CTS.

These include:

- **Genetic Predisposition:** Small bones or a small carpal canal increases the risk.
- **Hormonal Changes:** For women, hormones increase the chances of the syndrome; pregnancy and menopause can be particularly problematic.
- **Diseases:** Conditions like arthritis, lupus, diabetes and obesity can lead to narrowing of the canal.
- **Repetitive Motions:** Excessively doing activities like typing, using hand tools, gardening, golfing, sewing and massaging can repeatedly strain the area, causing localized inflammation and trauma.

COMMON CTS TREATMENT OPTIONS

There are a number of treatment options in wide use for the treatment of CTS. These include the use of wrist splints to brace the wrist in a neutral position to allow reduction in irritation of the area. You can also take a break from the activity that may be causing the CTS. But that is unrealistic if you depend on using your hands for a living.

Anti-inflammatory medications are also used to reduce pain and inflammation, as well as corticosteroids. However, these are not recommended for long-term use because of potentially serious side effects. Physical therapy and surgery round out the list of usual treatment options, but they offer only varying degrees of success.

SELF-ACUPRESSURE TREATMENT

In my clinical practice I developed a self-acupressure method that has proven successful in various degrees with my own clients and those of my colleagues. The theory is based on traditional Chinese medicine (TCM) and acupuncture. This philosophy takes into account not only the physical canal space but also the role of blood, lymph and muscle in the prevention and treatment of CTS.

In a nutshell, here is the technique you can use:

- Extend your forearm, wrist and palm muscles to stimulate blood flow and reduce muscle contraction pain and tightness.
- Press specific acupoints to remove energetic stagnations and promote free flow of qi or energy.
- Restore range of motion.

- Reduce inflammation, pain and stagnation in the carpal tunnel, hand, wrist and forearm.

Repeat this procedure several times a day for best results. If you are in an early stage of the condition, you get the best results. But even long-term sufferers can find relief.

EASY RELIEF FOR THE HEEL PAIN OF PLANTAR FASCIITIS

Heel pain affects millions of Americans annually. There are many reasons for its occurrence, including Achilles tendonitis and bone spurs; but the most common cause is plantar fasciitis. If not treated, plantar fasciitis can cause acute foot pain and affect the hips and back. But surgery or invasive procedures are not needed to relieve its symptoms. A combination of natural symptomatic relief methods and prevention techniques can go a long way and cost virtually nothing.

INFLAMED HEELS

Plantar fasciitis is inflammation of the plantar fascia ligament. This is the thick, fibrous band of tissue on the bottom of the foot that runs between the calcaneus (heel bone) and the toes. With each step or action of the foot, the ligament stretches. When plantar fascia becomes stressed, it develops tears that cause pain and swelling. The pain is most often felt under the heel bone.

COMMON SYMPTOMS

While generalized tenderness and pain are usually experienced under the heel, many people also experience stabbing and burning pain sensations. Pain is most severe in the morning, getting better as the day progresses and even better at night when you're off your feet. This symptomatic timeline occurs because the plantar fascia ligament becomes tight as we sleep. When we first awake and begin to walk, the taut band is painful. As the day progresses and blood moves throughout the body, allowing the muscles and ligaments to relax, the pain decreases. However, extended periods of walking or standing can cause the ligament to swell and become painful again.

PRIMARY CAUSES

There are quite a few things that can cause you to experience plantar fasciitis. Athletes and the elderly are most at risk, as are those whose job or vocation requires them to walk or stand for hours at a time.

Athletes place a good deal of stress on the ligament through the dynamic actions of their chosen sporting activities like running, jumping, twisting and dodging. Such repetitive stress over time can cause tears in the tissue that cause irritation, inflammation and pain.

The elderly are susceptible to developing tears in their plantar fascia for three reasons. As we age, we lose flexibility in our muscles and ligaments; but we usually don't alter our activities to compensate for this change. The tissues are also more susceptible to being overstressed as we age. And certain diseases common among older Americans, like diabetes and arthritis, cause plantar fasciitis through negative autoimmune responses, systemic inflammation and obstructed blood flow to the lower legs and feet.

IT'S THE SHOES

Wearing wrong-fitting shoes for work, play or social outings is also a common cause of heel pain from inflammation of the planter fascia. Wearing high heels, boots or other poor-fitting shoes causes issues with your gait, the distribution of weight over the heel and foot, stress to the tendons and ligaments, and tears in the ligaments.

Weight is another factor in heel and foot pain. Much of the weight you carry naturally or haul for work or during an activity is absorbed by the heel and distributed over the feet. Too heavy a load placed on your feet over a period of days or months or more can damage the plantar fascia. Pregnant women are also at risk for this same reason, although their extra weight is only temporary.

Finally, some people are born with a predisposition to stressing, irritating and tearing their plantar fascia because of abnormalities such as having flat feet, high arches, pronated feet and an abnormal gait. In these cases, like in athletic activities, over time, the plantar fascia is stressed and stretched past its ability to cope; and it succumbs to tears, inflammation and pain.

As can be seen from these examples, almost everyone is at risk for developing plantar fasciitis at some point in life. Many people have the misfortune of being at risk from several of the causes. The good news is that relief from symptoms is found in easy-to-do techniques and methods that require little to no cost, time or space.

NATURAL REMEDIES

The first line of care for an acute flare-up of plantar fasciitis is to stop your activity, seek some rest, take an over-the-counter anti-inflammatory (or a natural one like turmeric or arnica) and apply ice to reduce swelling and pain. The goal is to prevent the heel issue from recurring. Let's look at simple, natural ways to help.

- Stop all activities that cause or aggravate the condition for a period of time ample enough to begin the healing process.
- Apply ice as needed to reduce swelling and reduce pain so you can get through your day.
- Get ample rest to relax the area and for the body to process the inflammation and begin its repair.
- Stretch your calf muscles to take some of the stress off your Achilles tendon and off your foot. This can also help correct foot pronation and your gait.

- Massage your feet (top and bottom) and your calves to increase blood flow and reduce tension and stress in the area overall.
- Wear only proper-fitting and supportive shoes that plant you firmly on the ground and allow for the elastic movement of the plantar fascia. Don't rotate or tip your pelvis or low back in an effort to keep your posture erect. That means no high heels.
- If you have flat feet or high arches, see a podiatrist to inquire about having an orthotic insert made for your shoe or shoes to help provide the support you need to stop stressing your feet and to help distribute weight properly over the heel and foot.
- If you are overweight, you must change your eating and activity habits to shed those extra pounds. Not only are a sedentary lifestyle and a poor diet bad for your heart and health overall, but dropping pounds reduces the stress on your heels and helps prevent tears and inflammation of your plantar fascia.

PREVENTIVE MEDICINE

Prevention is always the best medicine. If you suffer from acute or chronic plantar fasciitis or generalized heel pain, take the necessary action to stop the things you are doing that cause it. Change your activities, switch shoes, lose weight, get more rest, use natural anti-inflammatory supplements, stretch and massage the area. Use an orthotic if you need one. If all this fails to bring relief in short order, then make an appointment with a podiatrist to have some tests and scans done to see if your heel pain is caused by something other than tears in the plantar fascia. But since plantar fasciitis is the most common cause of heel pain, give these remedies a shot to see how you can help yourself feel better.

VANQUISH JOINT PAIN ON THE CELLULAR LEVEL

Joint pain can be a life-wrecking experience. Pain is caused by many conditions, including arthritis, labrum tears, tight tendons, sprains, strains, dehydration and injury. For relief, many people turn to NSAIDs (nonsteroidal anti-inflammatories), analgesic drugs, MSM, glucosamine and chondroitin. Others use topical ointments like Sombra®, IcyHot®, BENGAY® and Biofreeze®. But there is another product on the market that is worth looking into: Celadrin®.

WHAT IS CELADRIN®?

Clinical studies show Celadrin® to be an effective anti-inflammatory compound that promotes healthy joint function. It increases joint flexibility and range of motion by lubricating the joint at a cellular level. Celadrin® is an ethylated esterified fatty acid derived from bovine tallow oil. Though it is similar to fish oil, it is made specifically to help joints through its action as a cellular lubricant.

HOW IT WORKS

Unlike NSAIDs, Celadrin® does not allow for better range of motion in the joints as a side effect of its pain relief and bodywide reduction of inflammation. Rather, it works to decrease inflammation specifically in the joints and lubricate their movement. It increases the fluids that cushion the space between the joint bones.

Because of its inflammation-reducing effects and lubricating actions, Celadrin® helps create an interior environment that allows the body to repair joints and adjacent tissues. It is reported to effect change at the cellular level, within the cell membranes themselves. It assists in the reduction and prevention of breakdown in joint cartilage.

THE STUDIES

Celadrin® has been scientifically studied for oral and topical efficacy. Findings have been published in such places as the *Journal of Rheumatology* and the *Journal of Strength and Conditioning Research*. In one double-blind, multi-center, placebo-controlled study, 64 participants (ages 37 to 77) took Celadrin® capsules daily for 68 days. Evaluated at days 30 and 68, the Celadrin® group reported greater flexibility and fewer aches. They were able to walk farther when compared to the placebo group.

Topical application of Celadrin® for 42 patients with osteoarthritis of the knee was studied at the University of Connecticut. Participants were evaluated before application of Celadrin® cream, 30 minutes after application, and again after twice-daily topical application for 30 days. Researchers in this study evaluated physical function, postural movement, range of motion and pain levels. Specifically, the study looked to evaluate real-world effects, including how long it took participants to "get up and go" from a chair, time in climbing stairs and improvements in knee mobility and endurance. When compared to the placebo cream group, 100% of those applying Celadrin® showed reduced pain and stiffness, better mobility and improved balance and strength.

The participants experienced a dramatic improvement in all aspects tested after only 30 minutes of applying the cream with cumulative beneficial effects occurring after 30 days.

MORE THAN A JOINT PAIN RELIEVER

There is one thing that arthritis, heart attacks, allergies, cancer, bowel diseases and Alzheimer's have in common: inflammation. The presence of inflammation can be felt and seen symptomatically when you suffer pain, heat, redness and swelling.

Inflammation is an essential component to fighting infection and repairing from injury. However, left unchecked, it wreaks havoc on the body. As a natural anti-inflammatory fatty acid compound, Celadrin® can help the body manage damaging symptoms through controlling inflammatory conditions. Studies have also shown it to be effective at reducing the effects of psoriasis.

THINGS TO CONSIDER

If you experience joint pain or inflammation of any kind not related to injury, please speak with your primary healthcare provider for advice. You need to know if the inflammation or pain is the result of a potentially serious medical issue. If so, you can get appropriate treatment. But if your pain is linked to inflammation, Celadrin® can help mitigate your problem while lubricating your joints and reducing pain. It helps the body heal.

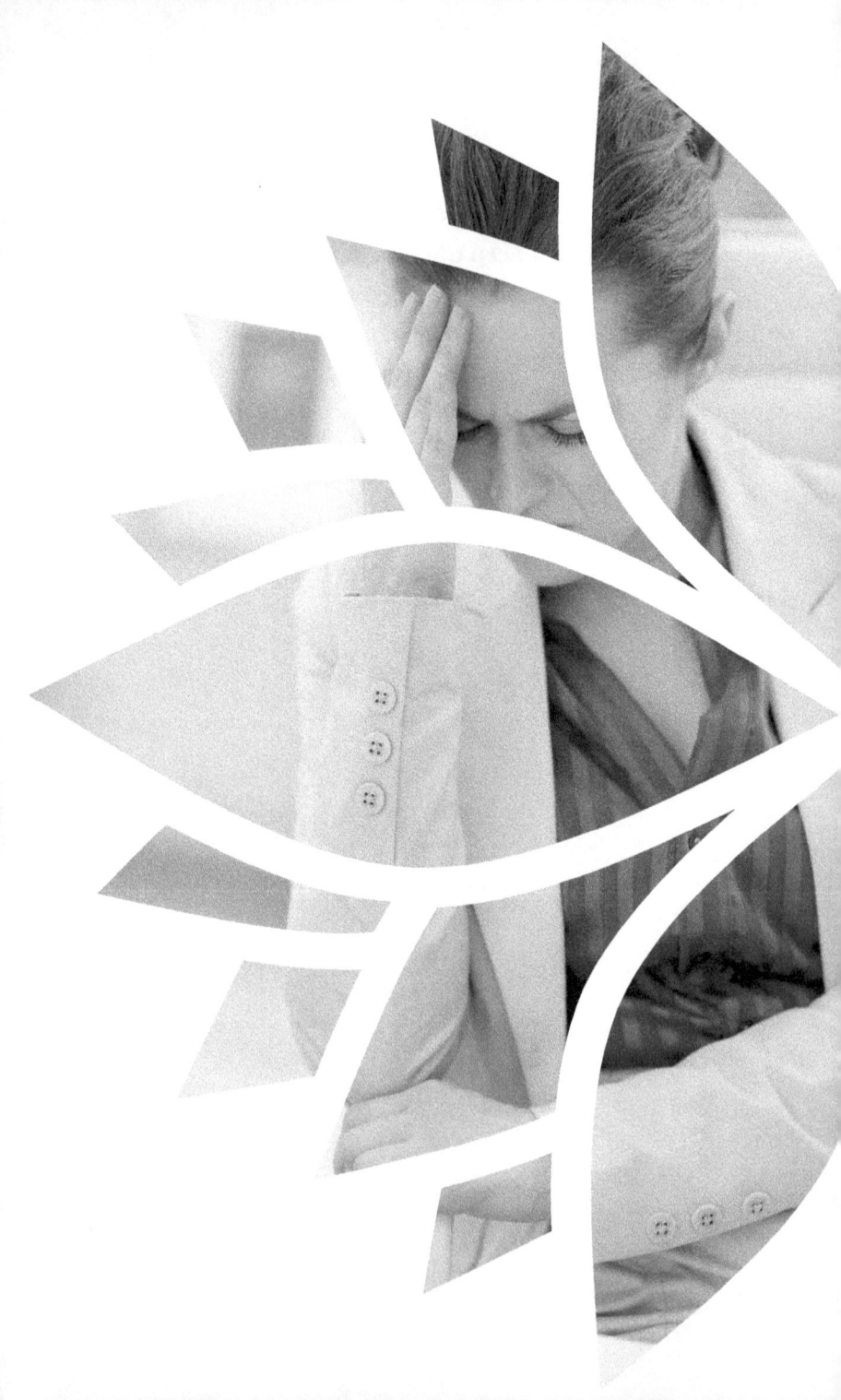

CHAPTER 10

REAL SOLUTIONS TO THE MIGRAINE PUZZLE

When I was very young I experienced something that can knock you flat on your back even as a full-grown adult:

Migraine headaches.

After becoming a medical practitioner, migraines were one of the first things I set out to help people overcome. Through my personal experience and years of helping patients, I have created both daily plans to prevent them, and self-care models for acute strikes.

Like everything related to health and wellness, I am not pro this and con that. I believe if it works, use it – but at the appropriate time.

If you can alter your sleep patterns to reduce sleep-deprivation headaches, that's easier, safer and less toxic than continuing to sleep fewer hours and taking an over-the-counter pain reliever the next day.

That's just one example, but I'm always on the lookout for new approaches to migraine and headache treatment.

Just the other day I came across a new intervention that I want to tell you about. But first, let me show you why and how you get migraines, and then we'll explore what you can do to stop them.

WHAT ARE MIGRAINES?

Headaches and migraines are not the same thing, exactly. A migraine is a type or classification of headache, but it's really a neurological disorder syndrome.

A syndrome is a collection of symptoms that you get stemming from a similar cause. Symptoms of migraine can include visual aura (bright lights, lines or distortion of sight), intense pain on one side of the head or behind one eye, nausea, vomiting, heightened sensitivity to light, smells, touch and sounds or vertigo-like dizziness.

Migraine attacks can last from several hours to several days. Some of my worst lasted nearly a week. And, they can be triggered by another headache type, or worsen with physical or psychological stress.

If you have migraines, you know that you can get a little stressed out and anxious wondering when you might have an attack… which itself might trigger a migraine.

Or you may have experienced depression and fatigue because of the extreme nature of the pain and suffering, and the life-altering nature of migraine attacks.

STEPS TOWARD A CURE

The only cure for migraines is to prevent them. This can be a bit tough because there are so many triggers.

Fortunately, I've helped countless people use many effective prevention models and treatments.

WHAT TO DO AT THE FIRST SIGN OF A MIGRAINE

If you haven't found a prevention model that works for you all the time, then it's important to recognize the signals your body sends that you're getting a migraine, and to take medication right away.

If you don't, you're leaving yourself open to experience the full force of the pain… and at that point, the medications are usually no longer effective.

Even showers, ice packs, analgesics and sleep don't seem to help. At this point many want to scrape their head on the bathroom tiles, or pray for mercy. When I was a kid, I wanted to hide in a dark corner…

SYMPTOM MASKING IS NOT PROBLEM SOLVING

While the Western scientific method views pain, illness and disease very specifically, Eastern systems do not. Western bioscience is based on a reductionist view of the body, finding the smallest thing responsible for a change and trying to adjust, fix or block it. In other words, if one is experiencing pain, this philosophy advocates taking a medication to block the pain receptors; problem solved. If you can't sleep, you're supposed to take a tablet to induce sleep. Again, problem solved. If you have diarrhea, drink or take something to halt the flow and that solves the problem.

Yet, health problems have never been solved using such methods. When a close friend of mine told me about "the worst headache in his life," he said it awakened him at 2AM and left him up all night in pain, scraping his head against the carpet to find relief. Eventually, he vomited. I'm not telling you that to gross you out, just to illustrate how bad it can get.

He told me the headache lasted three days and he ended up experiencing severe stomach pain, acid reflux, burning in his intestines and other problems from the amount of medicine he took to relieve the pain.

The pain meds did not work, as often happens, but he kept trying and eventually took too many, leading to a new and different collateral issue – GI discomfort.

He called me to ask why the medications had not worked and how such a headache can last for so long. My answer was simple, and it offered him a method to discover the root cause of his pain, which I am going to share with you now.

WHY THINGS WORK AND WHY THEY DON'T

When the body is off-kilter (not working at homeostasis), there is potential for a downward turn in health, reduced feeling of vitality and an increase in pain or other symptoms. Symptomatic treatment may, in fact, provide some temporary relief from a health issue, which may be much needed in the moment. However, many people tend to experience the same adverse health conditions again and again, at intervals or continuously throughout their lives. And it is not healthy or kind to the body to keep swallowing chemical pills and liquids for prolonged periods. In the short run, these solutions are powerful at getting over the hump, so to speak. But in the long run (and sometimes in the short run), they lead to a host of health problems like liver damage, heart disease, GERD, IBS, kidney dysfunction, chronic inflammation and rebound pain.

Masking the symptoms of pain, for example, will never prevent the pain from returning. Nor will it necessarily address the pain you may be experiencing. The example offered in my introduction shows that despite taking more painkillers than necessary, my friend suffered his headache in full force for several days. What's more, the overuse of pain meds led to a new rebound health issue within the digestive tract. This was followed by another issue: the dreaded "rebound" headache – a new headache is created as a reaction to the medication.

So the big question that puzzled my friend was: Why didn't the headache tablets take away his headache or reduce its pain? The answer is: Because they were not the right solution to the problem. While it may sound counterintuitive, just because a product or therapy is marketed to help relieve the symptoms of a headache, for example, does not mean it can actually do this all of the time. Why not? Because not every symptom (in this case a headache) is caused by the same thing every time it occurs.

Not all pain is the same. And not every product works for every type of pain. While ibuprofen is often successful in reducing inflammation, it does not help much when muscle spasm is an issue. Sometimes, pain is caused by inflammation; other times, it is triggered by muscle contraction.

In the case of contractions (tightness, trigger points), muscle relaxation is needed. This can be accomplished as a result of medication, but just as easily (and with less harm to the body) from massage, stretching and meditation.

ONE PROBLEM, MANY CAUSES

One of the tenets of traditional Chinese medicine (TCM) is that there are many causes of the same problem and that one cause can manifest in many ways. In other words, if 10 people suffer from migraine headaches and see a Western-trained healthcare provider, they may all receive the same prescription medication. After all, in the Western medical philosophy, symptoms of pain and poor health are labeled and the label (not the person) is treated. The label "migraine" is treated with certain drugs regardless of anything else going on in a person's body or life.

In TCM, if 10 people present with migraine headache, the practitioner will assess their overall health and mental state while taking into consideration lifestyle, diet, stress and sleep issues, to name a few. From this larger comprehensive and more holistic assessment, the TCM practitioner may find that while each of the 10 patients is experiencing what is labeled a "migraine," they all have different reasons. Therefore, their treatment will be different. Some will receive herbal therapy, others acupuncture, dietary therapy, massage or energy therapy. In other words, while each person is manifesting a headache, the cause of why or how the blood vessels changed is different and so then is the solution for each person.

UNDERSTAND YOUR PROBLEM TO HELP UNCOVER THE ROOT

So how can you uncover the root cause of your health issues to make better relief or therapeutic choices? The first thing is to discuss the potential causes of your issue with your primary healthcare provider. Knowledge is power, especially when it comes to taking control of your own health and wellness. Second, if you are a chronic headache sufferer, for example, then you can do some research online and easily find the common triggers for headaches.

You will find that headaches are commonly caused by exposure to chemical toxins in cleaning supplies, detergents and nitrates, as well as food preservatives, sugar, caffeine, fats, dairy products, red wine, citrus fruits and nightshade vegetables. It can also be linked to dehydration, lack of consistent sound sleep, lack of physical activity, muscle tension and stress. That's quite a list, and it is only a partial one.

Make a comprehensive list of what causes headaches and keep it handy. Every time you feel a headache, keep a journal of what you did, what you ate, your stress levels, your sleep time, the weather and so on. When you begin to reconcile the two lists, you will find the likely headache trigger or triggers appearing again and again. This is a pattern you can recognize. Your pattern causes your own bodily imbalance which, in turn, causes your symptom, which may be headaches. Like my friend, if you experience a prolonged headache and the solution you reach for does not work within a reasonable time, you must seek another solution. If the headache is caused by lack of sleep (which is quite common), then no amount of Advil® or Excedrin® will alleviate it. Only getting ample sleep, continuously, over a few days will.

OWN YOUR HEALTH

Your quality of life and state of health is personal and individual, and there is no one-size-fits-all approach that has proven effective or safe. Taking the wrong medication or seeing the wrong health practitioner for your health concerns will never help you. When you find something is not working, you must look for other solutions. And this process starts with a discussion with your healthcare provider and also with some personal research into your chronic conditions. If you can become familiar with the potential causes (triggers) of the headaches you experience and you can keep track of the ones presenting in your daily life, then you can be better equipped to find the correct and correlated solution.

If you have "the worst headache ever" and double doses of nonsteroidal anti-inflammatory drugs (NSAIDs) are not working, don't take more and expect relief. This only causes further health issues. Instead, try to uncover the root cause of your pain and then look for solutions that can safely and effectively address it.

MIGRAINE PAIN: STOPPING THIS GATEWAY TO A STROKE

If you've never had to go through the pain of a migraine headache, you should consider yourself lucky.

For those of us who have, we know migraine headaches as a painful and life altering condition. I know, because I suffered them almost daily for 30 years.

Every time they finally go away you think there's no way you can take that kind of pain again. And each time they come back you are on your back, lights off, ice packs, heat packs... and terrible pain in your stomach from the severity of the medication.

Inflammation, nausea, vomiting. Not to mention the changes in your visual field. These are known as aura, and here's something new about them.

Migraines have already been associated with heart attack. But new research links those who suffer migraine with aura to nearly double the risk of stroke.

That's why today I want to tell you how to slash that risk, and about another new treatment for migraine pain that could help you if you're suffering.

THE NATURE OF THE BEAST

Again, migraine headaches are vascular in nature. That means they are triggered by changes in the blood vessels in the brain. They are also associated with the trigeminal nerve, which wraps from the base of the skull around the sides of the head to the temple areas.

While the precise cause of migraine is not singular, there are many factors known to trigger them. Some of the more common triggers include humidity, air pressure, stress, lack of sleep or disturbed sleep and diets high in sugar, fat, preservatives, nitrates, MSG, alcohol, coffee and black tea.

Regardless of the trigger, classic migraines are pre-warned with visual aura and usually present with sensitivity to light, sound and smell and bouts of nausea and vomiting.

Research has shown that those who suffer migraines are at increased risk of heart attack and arterial claudication (leg pain due to poor circulation).

And recent studies and meta-analysis show a strong correlation between migraine and the most common form of stroke (roughly 85% of strokes are caused by blood clots in the brain).

WHY THE HUGE RISK TO YOUR BRAIN?

Loyola Medicine recently released results of a meta-analysis carried out by Loyola University Medical Center neurologists Michael Star, MD, and José Biller, MD They present three very significant findings:

1. Those who suffer migraine with aura are at nearly double the risk of stroke.
2. Migraine sufferers who smoke are at more than triple the risk of stroke.
3. Migraine sufferers who both smoke and use birth control are seven times more likely to suffer stroke.

Drs. Star and Miller dedicate an entire chapter to the association of stroke and migraine in their new book, *Headache and Migraine Biology and Management*, edited by Seymour Diamond of the National Headache Foundation.

After completing their meta-analysis, the researchers have proposed several possible explanations for the migraine-stroke association:

1. Migraine sufferers are more likely to have risk factors for cardiovascular disease, including low levels of "good" HDL cholesterol and high levels of C-reactive protein.
2. Specific genes may predispose people to suffer both migraines and stroke.
3. Medications to treat migraines may increase the risk of stroke.
4. A phenomenon that occurs during migraine aura, called cortical spreading depression, might trigger an ischemic stroke. A cortical spreading depression is a slowly propagated wave of depolarization, followed by depression of brain activity occurring during migraine aura. It includes changes in neural and vascular function.

Drs. Star and Biller conclude, *"...the research may point to stroke and migraine sharing a reciprocal causal relationship."*

The important thing here, then, is to reduce the incidence of migraine and to stop smoking and discontinue birth control (if possible) if you suffer migraine with aura.

Additionally, the severity and continuance of migraine can be greatly reduced with a new treatment.

IMAGE-GUIDED MIGRAINE TREATMENT

The Society of Interventional Radiology recently released data on their new treatment method for migraine headache. Clinicians at Albany Medical Center and the State University of New York Empire State College have used a treatment called image-guided, intranasal sphenopalatine ganglion (SPG) blocks.

That's a lot of science speak, but the goal is a simple one: to give patients enough ongoing migraine relief that they required less medication.

Lead study researcher Kenneth Mandato, MD, and team conducted a retrospective analysis of 112 patients suffering migraine or cluster headaches. According to Mandato, *"administration of lidocaine to the sphenopalatine ganglion acts as a 'reset button' for the brain's migraine circuitry."*

The treatment may seem like something not for the faint of heart, but if you've ever suffered the pain of a migraine, you'll do about anything to get rid of it. So I'll describe what the researchers did. They inserted a spaghetti-sized catheter through the nasal passages and administered 4% lidocaine to the sphenopalatine ganglion, a nerve bundle just behind the nose associated with migraines.

The results? Pain was cut in half.

Prior to treatment, patients reported an average pain score of 8.25. After treatment those scores were halved, averaging at 4.10. What's more, after treatment nearly 90% of patients reported needing less or no migraine medication for ongoing relief. For anyone who has or does suffer migraine, these results are significant and promising for pain relief.

While the new treatment method is no cure for migraine, it does offer promise in the relief of chronic migraine pain that can be crippling and life-changing. And once there is a break in the pain cycle, migraine sufferers can stop chasing relief and taxing their bodies with drugs and begin the path of prevention.

I've written about natural means of migraine relief and prevention many times. The essential thing is to reduce pain when the migraine is in control, and to prevent the migraine from triggers every other day. By preventing the trigger you can not only live a better life, but greatly reduce your risk for stroke and heart disease.

I'd like to share a few more with you now.

AVOID TOXIC WATER BOTTLES AND PACKAGING

Researchers Nancy Berman and Lydia Vermeer at Kansas University (KU) Medical Center had a hypothesis they wanted to test. Since more women than men get migraines, and they often are related to the menstrual cycle, perhaps hormones play a key role in migraines. They also wondered if bisphenol A (BPA), a hormone-disrupting chemical used to make plastic firm, might play a part. BPA leaks into food or drink from food and beverage containers. When you consume BPA, the chemical acts like estrogen.

Does BPA, then, also trigger migraines?

To put this hypothesis to the test, they injected lab rats with BPA and found that, in fact, the BPA activated estrogen receptors. The lab animals also displayed significantly worse headache symptoms than animals not exposed to BPA.

"We're hypothesizing that people with migraines do not have more BPA in their system, but that they're more sensitive to BPA," Vermeer said. "Many people with migraines are more sensitive to changes in things like estrogen."

While the Food and Drug Administration (FDA) has declared BPA to be safe in low levels, it has also expressed concern about deleterious effects on the brain, behavior and in the prostate health of young children and fetuses. As such, the FDA has banned the use of BPA from baby bottles and drink nipples.

Hmmm, sounds "unsafe" to me! To boot, Canada, France and China have actually banned BPA from many consumer applications.

BPA is found in water bottles, including those with recycle codes of #3 and #7, and also in the lining of many canned goods. The problem is that one of the preventive measures of migraines is to drink plenty of water. So that's a real problem.

The new solution: Drink filtered water out of a glass container, glass or plastic bottle that is marked "BPA Free." I do. And while we don't yet have clear proof of a human reaction, as we do with rats, it takes no money and little effort to prevent a migraine by changing the type of vessel from which we consume our water. So the good news here is that we are now aware of another potential migraine trigger (BPA) and we can easily avoid it by purchasing canned goods and plastic contained food and beverages marked BPA Free or indicating recycling code #2.

LED LIGHTS TO THE RESCUE

The end of incandescent light bulb use in the United States draws nigh. As part of the Energy Independence and Security Act of 2007 (originally called the Clean Energy Act of 2007), light bulb manufacturers must produce 40 watt bulbs that only draw 10.5 watts of energy, and 60 watt bulbs that draw only 11 watts of energy. The result is compact fluorescent bulbs (CFLs) and LED lights.

What's this got to do with migraines?

For starters, it is known that flickering lights can trigger migraines and seizures. One theory is that migraine headaches are subdural or deep seizures. Mark Green, MD, director of the Center for Headache and Pain Medicine at the Icahn School of Medicine at Mount Sinai, told FOX News that, *"most migraine sufferers enjoy incandescent lighting, since it doesn't produce any flickering sensations and has a nice warm feel. But with this change, it's going to be harder for individuals to avoid fluorescent lights."*

The good news is that LED lights, although more expensive than CFLs and other types of bulbs, are not constructed of filaments. Therefore, there is zero flickering. (The movements of electrons in a semiconductor triggers illumination.)

Now, with LED technology, people can conserve energy, light a room and do something proactively to avoid another migraine trigger.

FIRST-EVER FDA-APPROVED MIGRAINE DEVICE

According to a recent press release, the FDA has allowed marketing of the Cerena Transcranial Magnetic Stimulator (TMS), the first device to relieve pain caused by migraine headaches that are preceded by an aura (a visual, sensory or motor disturbance that immediately precedes the onset of a migraine attack).

The Cerena TMS is a prescription device used after the onset of pain associated with migraine headaches preceded by an aura. Simply hold the devise to the back of the head and press a button, and a pulse of magnetic energy stimulates the brain's occipital cortex. Trials show this can stop or greatly decrease symptoms of migraine.

The FDA reviewed a randomized control clinical trial of 201 patients who had mostly moderate to strong migraine headaches and who had auras preceding at least 30% of their migraines. Of the study subjects, 113 recorded treating a migraine at least once when pain was present. Analysis of these 113 subjects was used to support marketing authorization of the Cerena TMS for the acute treatment of pain associated with migraine headache with aura.

The study showed that nearly 38% of subjects who used the Cerena TMS when they had migraine pain were pain-free two hours after using the device, compared to about 17% of patients in the control group. After 24 hours, nearly 34% of the Cerena TMS users were pain-free compared to 10% in the control group.

If this product really works as claimed, it could be a game-changer in the lives of millions. Visit this website for more information: http://www.fda.gov/NewsEvents/Newsroom/PressAnnouncements/ucm378608.htm

THE BEST NUTRIENTS AND VITAMINS FOR MIGRAINE RELIEF

Americans spend millions of dollars annually on analgesics, anti-inflammatories, beta blockers, calcium channel blockers, triptans and other medical chemicals to help stave off and reduce the pain and other symptoms associated with headaches.

While drugs, both prescribed and over-the-counter, are the most popular remedy for headache and migraine, they may not be the most effective; and they certainly are not without side effects. Natural vitamins and nutritional supplements, in some cases, have been shown to be just as effective (and some more effective) than their lab-produced counterparts. Here, we'll look at those proven to be most effective.

Supplementation that combines vitamins B6, B12 and folate (the active form of folic acid) has been shown to be effective in the treatment of migraines that are accompanied with aura.

Studies show that those who experience the so-called "classic migraine" (that is, the migraine that follows a visual aura) have elevated levels of homocysteine. Homocysteine is an amino acid in the blood that, when it rises too high, can lead to a host of health issues, including blood vessel blockages and migraine headaches.

Levels of homocysteine rise when it is not metabolized properly; this can be caused by low levels of certain B vitamins and folic acid. Studies have shown that in addition to diets high in these vitamins, or merely supplementing with B12, B6 and folate, you can help the body process metabolize homocysteine and bring it down to a normal level, thus helping prevent classic migraines.

A blood test can determine if high homocysteine is causing your migraines.

VITAMIN BENEFITS

These supplements can help lower your migraine risk:

- **Vitamin B6 (Pyridoxine):** Works to stave off migraines by supporting a broad number of activities in your nervous system, breaking down sugars and starches, and metabolizing homocysteine. In addition to taking a supplement, food sources include: avocado, bananas, beans, sunflower seeds, spinach, potatoes, tuna, cod, halibut, liver, chicken, turkey and eggs.

- **Vitamin B12:** Supports the proper development of nerve cells and red blood cells and helps prevent anemia while helping metabolize protein, carbohydrates, fat and homocysteine levels in the blood. Cyanocobalamin is a lab-made version of this vitamin that has shown to be effective, via pill and injection. In addition, the following foods are good sources of B12: yogurt, grass-fed beef and cow's milk, lamb, shellfish, salmon, sardines and scallops.

- **Vitamin B2 (Riboflavin):** Supports the production of cellular energy. B2 is an antioxidant that helps protect cells from free-radical oxygen damage and is a key component in the process of converting food to energy. As a supplement taken for three months at 400 mg per day, studies show it to reduce migraine onset by 50% in more than half of the people who take it. In addition to fortified grains, breads and cereals, riboflavin is found in lean meats, eggs, grass-fed cow's milk, yogurt, collard greens and other green leafy vegetables, nuts, legumes and cremini mushrooms.

- **Folic Acid/Folate (a B vitamin):** Helps metabolize homocysteine, supports the production of red blood cells and proper nerve function. Helps stave off some cancers, stroke, heart attack, anemia and migraine. In addition to supplements and fortified breads and cereals, good sources of folic acid include: beans (lima, pinto, navy, garbanzo), lentils, spinach, collard greens and turnip greens.

- **Magnesium:** Vital to health, as it plays important roles in a wide array of physiological processes. It is absorbed in the gastrointestinal tract (more when there is less fecal matter in it) and helps facilitate the absorption of calcium. In addition to pill and powder supplements, magnesium is naturally found in foods like seeds (sesame, sunflower), nuts (cashews, almonds), spices, meat, dairy products, green leafy vegetables (Swiss chard, spinach), tea, coffee, cocoa, black beans and halibut. Your body needs a certain amount every day; if you take too much, you will experience diarrhea.

- **Feverfew (Tanacetum parthenium):** Has been studied more than any other supplement for its effects on migraine. It has been shown to help reduce the frequency and severity of migraines in those who take 100 mg daily. Feverfew works by relaxing blood vessels and decreasing inflammation, thereby improving blood circulation in the brain.

- **Butterbur (Petasites hybridus):** A perennial shrub effective for people suffering migraine (without aura) when taken for four months at 75 mg twice daily. A 2004 study showed the best response after three months with a 58% reduction in attacks. A significant

71% of the nearly 250 people in the study responded positively to the supplement.

- **Omega-3 Fish Oils:** One of the most powerful and natural anti-inflammatories that have been shown to reduce the frequency, duration and severity of migraines. The three fatty acids in fish oil are known as ALA, DHA and EPA. Taking a combined dose of 1,000 mg daily can help with a host of issues, including headache and migraine.
- **CoQ10 (Coenzyme Q10):** Antioxidant produced by the body.

Aids in boosting cellular activity by taking part in the creation of ATP (adenosine triphosphate), the major source of cellular energy. A daily regimen of 200 mg has been shown to help energy levels. CoQ10 has been shown to help reduce the onset of migraine. The best food sources include salmon, tuna, organ meats and whole grains.

GREAT METHODS

Diet and supplementation are two great ways to get enough of the key vitamins and nutrients that are essential to help prevent, delay and reduce the frequency, duration and intensity of headaches (especially migraines).

I will conclude with advice from the New York Headache Center: *"The efficacy of some non-pharmacologic therapies appears to approach that of most drugs used for the prevention of migraine and tension-type headaches. These therapies often carry a very low* risk of serious side effects and frequently are much less expensive than pharmacologic therapies."

Safer and cheaper are always good things when it comes to quality of life and pain reduction.

CONTROLLING HEADACHE TRIGGERS

It is important to know a headache is not a disease; it is a symptom. Something or several things are needed to trigger a headache. Thus, while taking pain medication can certainly decrease the pain or other symptoms, they will not prevent the triggers from causing the headache. Controlling triggers leads to prevention of headaches.

Let's look at these now.

LIFESTYLE IS THE MAIN CULPRIT

When considered as a whole, the majority of things that cause or trigger headaches are the result of our lifestyles. When we choose to indulge in the foods, beverages and activities that are known triggers of headaches, we, therefore, choose to give ourselves a headache.

We then choose to take a pain-relieving medication to stop the headache, instead of changing our behaviors that maintain our unhealthy lifestyle. That may sound rough, but it is true. And believe me, having suffered excruciating headaches for decades, I know that we don't feel like headaches are a choice.

And sometime they are not. But for the common headaches not related to diseases or tumors or traumatic injury, the prevention of them is a choice worth choosing.

So how does lifestyle trigger headaches? In many ways, all of them relate to our daily choices and behaviors.

Most headaches can be controlled for as long as we choose a proactive approach rather than a reactive one. Lifestyle triggers include the duration and quality of our sleep, our work methods, exercise habits, emotional states and stress-relieving abilities. Other triggers include our diet and our home and work environments.

Let's look at these a bit more.

Digestion: This is related to your quality and state of health. Poor digestion is often the result of poor health practices. For example, constipation and a slow digestive tract are known headache triggers. The putrid waste is made to remain in the body too long, becomes toxic and partially enters the bloodstream. It then puts pressure on the liver to work overtime to clear toxins that keep circulating.

Diet: Digestive issues can be caused by eating a poor diet that includes things like too much fatty, fried and greasy items; too much sugar and simple carbohydrates; too many nitrates and MSG (found in hot dogs, luncheon meats); gluten (wheat, barley and rye products); and too much dairy (which is often fatty and also provides an environment for bacteria and sinus inflammation).

Moreover, drinking ample water is essential for better health. Beverages like coffee, tea, beer, wine and alcohol are diuretics that promote sweating and urination. These cause dehydration: The fluids needed for the kidney and other body functions to work properly are not replenished with water. Even a good diet of whole grains, fruits and vegetables can lead to digestive issues if one does not consume more water than diuretic beverages each day.

Sleep: Both sleeping too long and not long enough can trigger headaches. We need on average 7.5 hours of sound, quality sleep each night, which includes REM (rapid eye movement) time.

However, many of us cannot get this because of work/life schedule overload, too much extraneous noise, body pains that wake us, too much caffeine or exercise in the evening, a mind racing with stressful or anxious thoughts or having to get up several times to urinate.

But sleep is essential to well-being overall and to pain relief in general. This is the time the body shuts down its active mode and goes into repair mode. Stress hormones are metabolized during sleep. If your daily life is full of stress and those stress hormones are raging through your body causing digestive issues, tight shoulders and tension and anxiety or depression, not getting enough sleep on top of those problems can inflict great pain. Lack of sleep and stress are also both independently tied to high-risk premature mortality. It is essential that you choose to sleep well each night, in whatever way you can. Choose it and plan for it. So many chronic headaches can be avoided by adjusting your sleep pattern.

Oxygen: Mild oxygen deprivation is one of the hidden causes of pain and especially headache. Stress, anxiety and worry are all things that can lead to oxygen deprivation. It only takes a very small reduction in the amount of oxygen in the blood for pain to manifest.

Oxygen is among the essential elements needed to sustain life. It is life-providing and is needed for cellular respiration and metabolism. However, a lack of exercise, poor diet, stress, tight muscles, mental strain and improper breathing can decrease the amount of oxygen in the body. That can create pain and a weakening of the immune system. Sinus infections, inflamed mucus membranes, stuffy nose and a face pressed into a pillow while sleeping can all cause a mild deprivation of oxygen that can trigger a headache. To maintain your oxygen level, practice deep breathing, clear the nasal passages, eat whole foods and exercise to keep up your oxygen.

Stress: The problem of stress is that it sneaks up on you. Then, when you feel it, you may have already triggered headaches and heart disease. Stress hormones promote systemic inflammation, constricting blood flow, which restricts oxygen transport. Stress tightens the shoulders and neck and causes tension headaches. Stress dumps fight-or-flight hormones into the bloodstream that are often not metabolized and lead to pain and disease.

Stress can lead to digestive issues and sleep deprivation. All of this means headaches! Learn methods to reduce your stress, and you can control for its many headache triggers.

The migraine situation is really a puzzle in need of solving. And there is just so much to it, in addition to the numerous other types of headaches that need addressing.

The information in this chapter is the 'essence' of migraine relief and prevention. But if you still need more help, as many chronic sufferers do, you can learn to master your migraines and headaches in my forthcoming book, Headaches Relieved (coming Winter 2016 from Tambuli Media). It shares my 40 year battle with these monsters and the program I developed to rid the forever. Visit www.TambuliMedia.com for updates!

SPRAY AWAY MIGRAINE PAIN?

Without any outside funding, Dr. Kenneth Mandato and associates at the Albany Medical Center in Albany, NY, have come a long way to helping relieve migraine pain, severity and occurrence.

They've discovered a minimally invasive treatment using a type of "migraine spray." As you're reading this, they will have just presented the findings of their independent study at the annual meeting of the Society of Interventional Radiology in Atlanta, GA.

From there they seek peer-review in journal publication. Thanks to their news release, we don't have to wait so long to hear first news of their findings and their product.

The first thing I noticed is that the study for migraine reduction and prevention was not done by neurologists or by Big Pharma. Dr. Mandato and his team of radiologist partners carried it out.

Their new procedure "significantly alleviates" the pain associated with migraine.

It works very simply and non-invasively by spraying a local anesthetic called - (Xylocaine) directly on the nerves located inside the nasal cavity.

To administer the Lidocaine solution, researchers inserted a small catheter into the nasal passages of each of the 112 patient participants. All 112 participants were previously identified as being affected by cluster headaches, and their migraine symptoms and pain levels were assessed.

Researchers delivered a dose of the solution to the cluster of nerves located at the back of the nasal cavity, known as the Meckel's ganglion. There nerves are associated with the trigeminal nerve, which is now believed to be largely associated with headaches, both general and migraine.

The researchers believe that the Lidocaine somehow "short-circuits this neural highway's pathway associated with recurrent headaches or migraines."

It must work, because a single treatment reduced pain levels of a migraine episode from a self-reported 8 (out of 10) to a 4 (out of 10). What's more, the 35% pain reduction lasted a full month after the treatment.

In fact, 94% of the people in the study found fast and lasting pain relief, which is a very strong indicator of good things to come.

If you've ever needed to have an analgesic injection for migraines, then the news most promising about this treatment is that you won't have to worry anymore about toxicity that can harm to the liver, kidneys and G.I. tract.

And at some point, you might be able to have a spray bottle that you use maybe twice a year, and carry with you for emergencies.

Please use the protocols I outlined above and use the one that works best for you.

REFERENCES:

http://www.physiciansnews.com/2015/03/02/nerve-treatment-via-nose-shows-promise-against-migraines/

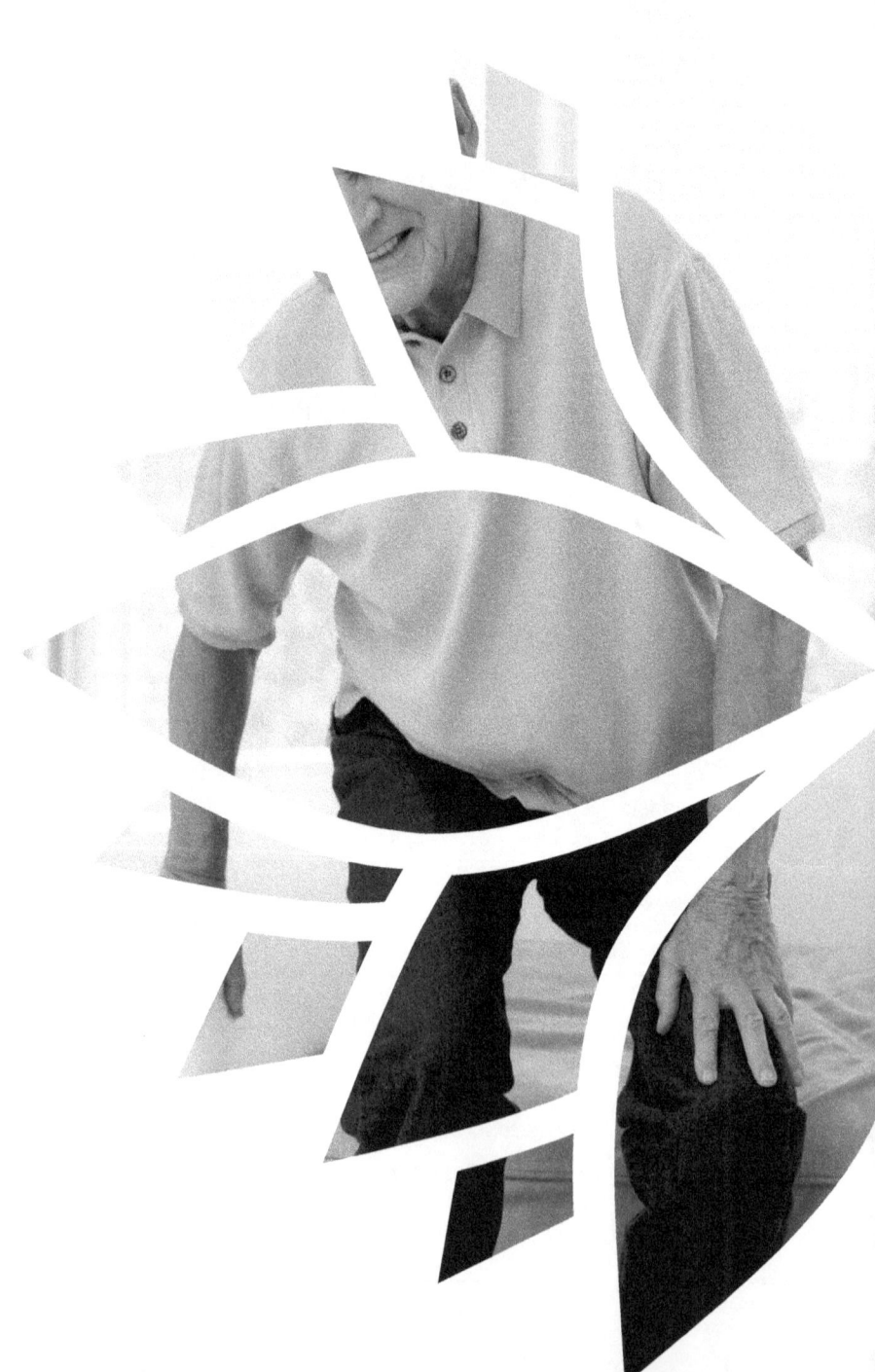

CHAPTER 11

REVERSING ARTHRITIS

TOP 10 ARTHRITIS MISTAKES

*M*aking mistakes is OK when dealing with health and trying to create a better quality of life.

But when you don't realize you are making mistakes, serious problems occur that put success out of reach.

This is a serious issue in the 10 most common mistakes people make when dealing with arthritis.

MISTAKE #1
WAITING TOO LONG TO ADDRESS ARTHRITIS

Even though there is no cure for arthritis, once you have been diagnosed, you must become proactive in managing, treating and slowing its progression. Reduction of symptoms and changes in lifestyle are essential from the start. Waiting too long to do something about arthritis is one of the biggest mistakes; it allows the condition to entrench itself in the body, to progress and to wreak havoc. There is no time like the present: Go ahead and make the decision to begin the rest of your life today by taking control of your arthritis.

MISTAKE #2
UNDERGOING ARTHROSCOPIC SURGERY

Plenty of research indicates without doubt that arthroscopic surgery, to "repair" arthritic joints and the space between them does not work. When it comes to fixing your arthritic condition, it is a mistake to go ahead with physician-recommended arthroscopic surgery. Given the number of years this practice has been in place, I can understand why this doesn't seem like a mistake, but it is. So if your primary care physician or orthopedic specialist suggests you have this procedure, please say, "No, thank you."

MISTAKE #3
AVOIDING EXERCISE, BEING SEDENTARY

I know when you are in pain, it is difficult to do what you used to do, and it takes serious effort to get up and keep moving. But it is a mistake to allow the symptoms of arthritis to keep you from enjoying a vibrant life. In fact, immobility and a sedentary lifestyle are contraindicated when it comes to arthritis. Physical activity lubricates the joints, maintains their range of motion, improves blood flow and stabilizes the muscles around arthritic joints. All of this reduces inflammation and pain as long as the exercise is within a range that you can perform without injury or further damage to your joints.

MISTAKE #4
ASSUMING IF YOU ARE "PHYSICALLY FIT" AND "EAT RIGHT" YOU WON'T GET ARTHRITIS

The physically fit and active among us are great at creating a worldview and building a lifestyle around being healthy, fit and vibrant. I would like active people to know that they are not safe from arthritis. You see, a condition like rheumatoid arthritis can come on at any time and for various unknown reasons; it is a result of an autoimmune disorder that has nothing to do with how physically fit you may be. And people who train hardest, run most intensely and jump the most over prolonged periods are most susceptible to osteoarthritis. They are at the highest risk for wearing down joints and damaging the cartilage between them.

A look at the people being treated at a physical therapy center shows this to be true. Anyone can suffer arthritis, not just the sedentary and sick. It is a mistake to think otherwise.

MISTAKE #5
NOT BELIEVING DIET AND NUTRITION PLAY A MAJOR ROLE IN ARTHRITIS

One of the key components of osteoarthritis prevention and reversal is embracing an organic, nutrient-dense diet and taking nutritional supplements to reduce symptoms and shore up wellness.

Our bodies are created from the stuff we eat. The quality of our cells and blood and tissues derive from the quality of our nutritional intake. Taking natural supplements to reduce inflammation and ease pain and improve joint motility is always easier on the body than taking artificial drugs. Don't fall victim to diet and nutrition mistakes. Instead, put nutritionally dense food into your body.

MISTAKE #6
THINKING MEDICAL SPECIALISTS HAVE ALL THE ANSWERS

Americans are taught to believe in a healthcare system that incorporates two practitioner categories: generalists and specialists. When it comes to arthritis, the specialist is usually an orthopedist or immunologist. In either case, it is a mistake to think these people have all the answers; they don't. Yes, they are highly educated in their specific field of treatment, but they are often ignorant of the available natural and holistic options. Oftentimes, they dismiss such options as so much hocus-pocus. It is important to note, however, that a medical specialist may have the right option for you. So keep an open mind in all cases and do look for multiple opinions and resources when considering the path you will take on your road to a better life.

MISTAKE #7
NOT GIVING NATURAL THERAPIES ENOUGH TIME TO WORK

Natural therapies, like herbal remedies, supplements, dietary changes, energy medicine and manual therapies that gently work the energy lines (meridians), the soft tissue and the skeletal system, are effective. As a matter of fact, they work very well, but only when given the time to do their job. They are gentle and take time to correct the imbalances within the body that cause arthritis or allow the condition to continue on its destructive course. Please do not give up on natural therapies and solutions. It is a mistake just to "try" them for a short period, or even a single time, and say they don't work because they didn't meet your expectation of immediate relief.

MISTAKE #8
CONTINUING ON A TREATMENT PLAN THAT'S NOT WORKING

If you do give a natural remedy the time necessary to work as it should, and it falls short for you or does not seem to help you, then it is a mistake to keep doing it. Additionally, continuing to take a medication to mask arthritic symptoms without altering the condition in a positive way is a mistake; discontinue it. Move on to the next therapy and find the mix of products, treatments and practices that, when combined, do what you need them to. Everyone reacts differently to therapies.

MISTAKE #9
BELIEVING THERE ARE NO MORE OPTIONS LEFT

Believing there are no options left – that you have exhausted all options within the medical profession for arthritis relief – is a mistake. There are many causes and triggers for arthritis and its symptoms. And the good news is that within the treasure chest of alternative medicine and holistic therapies are hundreds of options that can work for you. There is no one-size-fits-all approach to arthritis.

MISTAKE #10
FAILING TO TAKE PERSONAL CONTROL OF YOUR SITUATION

No one cares about your arthritic condition as much as you do. You are the one suffering, not others, so to rely on others to take care of your condition is a big mistake. You must take personal control of your arthritis. You are the only one who can change your lifestyle, removing the things that negatively impact your health and wellness. It is only you who can eat right and take supplements and administer pain relieving creams and gels. It is only you who can stretch, walk, exercise and meditate.

Why do I call this chapter "Reversing Arthritis"? Because it is excerpted from my ground-breaking book, *Arthritis Reversed*. This book details all aspects of arthritis and how you can reverse some of the damage caused by arthritis, reduce the symptoms, and prevent it from worsening. If you or someone you love has arthritis, visit TambuliMedia.com for free additional articles and to grab your copy of *Arthritis Reversed*.

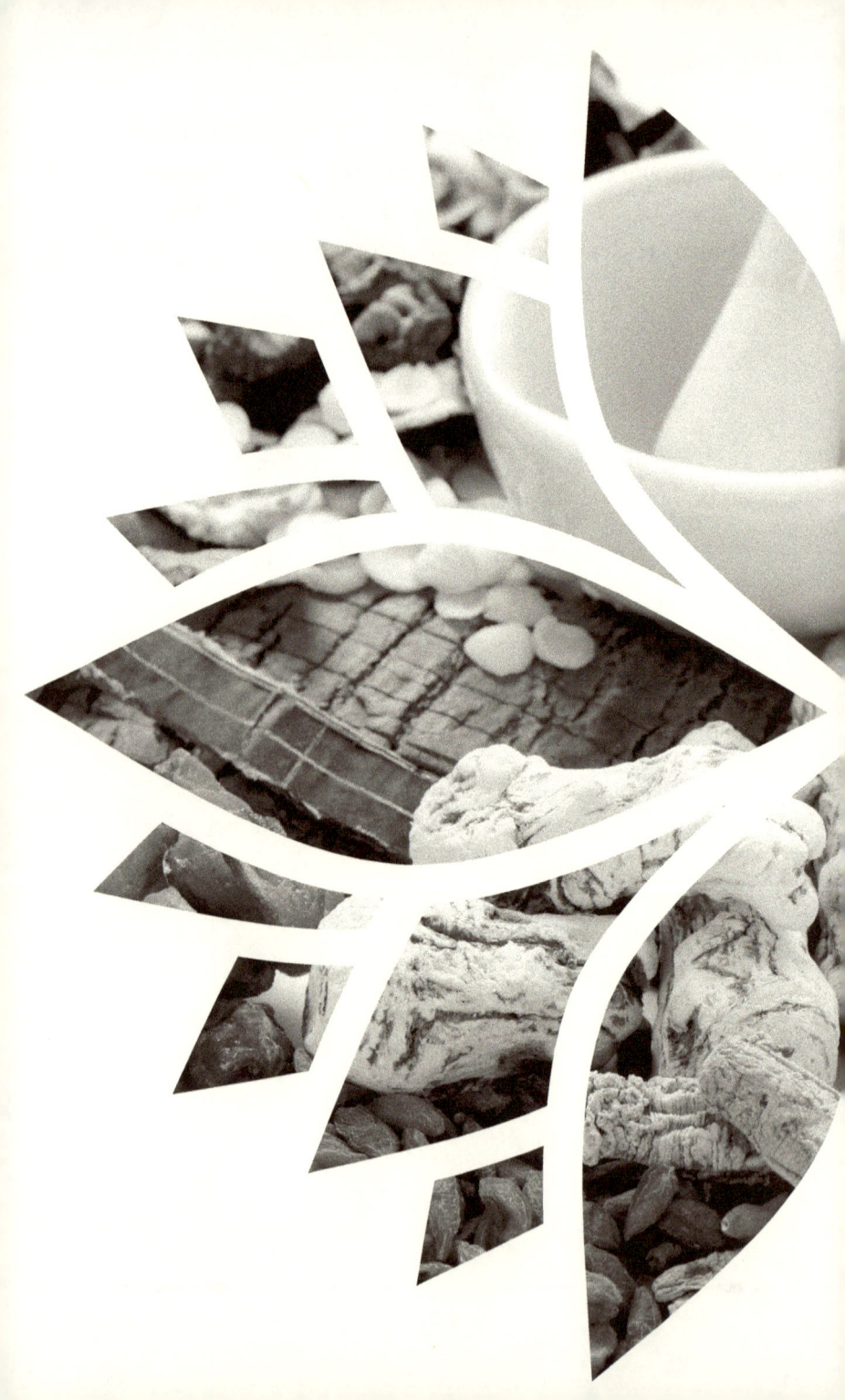

CHAPTER 12

CHINESE MEDICINE FOR PHYSICAL INJURIES

Every day people experience pain and physical injury from simple things. You can develop a stiff neck from sleeping wrong or a twisted ankle from a wrong step in sports or suffer broken bones from accidents.

Many of these – what I call "ordinary life pains and strains" – are not serious and do not require serious medical attention. But when left untreated, or if treated improperly, they can become chronic. One of the best overall modalities I have found to work well for many forms of physical trauma (e. g., pain, inflammation, bruising and strains) is traditional Chinese medicine (TCM).

TCM dates back thousands of years and has many different modalities that it uses to treat different forms of physical trauma. I was recently consulting with my friend and colleague Dr. Dale Dugas who specializes in making herbal formula, teas and topical liniments for physical trauma and here's what I have learned from him regarding the best forms of TCM for treating physical injury.

THE DIFFERENT WAYS IN WHICH TCM TREATS TRAUMA

Acute injuries typically manifest with moderate to severe pain, swelling, redness and heat. This is usually localized in the area that has been injured. Herbs can be applied externally to help reduce inflammation, decrease swelling and help deal with pain. These herbs are usually "cooling" and "moving" in their nature. You can prepare an oil based balm/paste with these herbs. They are applied to the injured area and covered with gauze and used for the first 24 hours to help reduce pain and swelling. Other herbs (whether in raw form or prepared as pills/capsules), can be taken to help deal with the swelling and pain caused by the trauma.

Other practitioners use a medicated plaster, which has herbs processed into the adhesive. These plasters are then applied to the affected area, and typically will be left on for three to 12 hours. The herbs in the adhesive help to reduce pain, increase circulation and help with increasing the blood flow to the injured area. Usually these types of plasters are used after the initial swelling has decreased.

Herbal liniments called Dit Da Jow (literally, Fall Strike Alcohol) are also used. The liquid made from herbs steeped into alcohol is applied to the area affected. Formulas with cooling herbs can be used to help reduce the initial swelling of an acute injury, but usually liniments are used in a manner similar to applying and using a plaster – i. e., after the swelling has decreased would this modality be used on an injury.

"HANDS-ON" TREATMENT METHODS

Acupuncture points can be stimulated with needles or finger pressure to help reduce swelling, pain and increase blood circulation in the area affected. Tui Na is a form of therapeutic massage that is used in TCM. After the swelling has decreased, medicated oil can be used to help increase blood circulation as well as a skin lubricant, and the affected area is worked on to help increase blood circulation as well as work out the fluids that have collected there due to the initial swelling from the injury.

METHODS TO USE IN THE HEALING PROCESS

Depending on the severity of the injury and the amount of heat and swelling at the affected area, most practitioners agree that one has to deal with the heat, pain and swelling immediately.

Modern use of ice was not utilized in China, as many would say the use of "ice was for dead people."

Herbs and balms/plasters can be applied quickly and easily, in or outside of a TCM clinic. These can easily be carried around in a first aid kit. Some TCM practitioners will bleed distal acupuncture points to affect an immediate healing response to an acute injury. This should only be done in a sterile setting, and not by a person looking for self-care.

The usual situation is that people do not come into TCM clinics with acute injuries, they come in after the initial 24-48 hour period and have mild to moderate swelling and an increase in pain. If the initial heat and swelling has been reduced, TCM practitioners typically start to work on increasing blood circulation in the affected area. Warming and pain-reducing herbs/liniments can be used to help increase blood flow.

What about chronic injuries?

Chronic injuries can be stubborn as they have been around for a period of time. One could use a hot external liniment or a strong internal formula to help increase blood flow, help open the acupuncture channels and reduce pain.

Here are some of the most-used herbs for different forms of physical injury or trauma.

- **Inflammation:** Bo He (mint), Chuan Xiong (Lovage Root), Mu Dan Pi (Peony Tree Root Bark), Ru Xiang (Frankincense), Bai Zhi (Angelica Root).
- **Pain:** Yan Hu Sou (Corydalis Root), Bai Shao (Peony Root), Bai Zhi (Angelica Root), Chai Hu (Buplerum root), Hai Feng Teng (Kadsura Pepper Stem), Mo Yao (Myrrh).
- **Bruising:** Chi Shao (Red Peony Root), Dang Gui Wei (Chinese Angelica Root), Hong Hua (Safflower).

- **Tendonitis:** Xu Duan (Dipsacus Root), Mu Gua (Chinese Quince Fruit), Shen Jin Cao (Clubmoss).

PROS AND CONS OF USING PLASTERS, DIT DA JOW AND HERBAL PILLS.

The biggest benefit of using trauma plasters is their ease of use. They are like bandages: You can store them anywhere. All you have to do is peel off the backing and stick them over the injury site. The only drawback is for people that are hairy. Removal could be a little painful and you will lose some body hair in the process.

Dit da jow liniments are great in that you will not lose body hair. The liquid is applied and rubbed into the injury site until it is fully absorbed dermally. The liquids can stain clothing so be careful. Some liniments are very odiferous and your co-workers might think you own a spice house. Patent medicines are herbs that are ground and pressed into tablets and rolled into tiny round pills. They are easy to store and have on your person or in your first aid kit. The only drawback is you have to ingest the pills, then digest them and then have your body figure out what to do once your body has recognized the herbs.

MAKE YOUR OWN DIT DA JOW LINIMENT.

Making a basic jow liniment is easy. You can take Hung Hua (Safflower) 18 grams, Ru Xiang (Frankincense), Mo Yao (Myrrh) both 18 grams, Xu Duan (Dipsacus Root) 18 grams, and Shen Jin Cao (Clubmoss) 18 grams and add this to a half gallon up to a gallon of vodka in a glass container. Do not waste your money on high-end alcohol; store-brand vodka is perfectly fine. Add these herbs, whether whole or cut up into big chunks, into the medium. You can agitate it daily for one week and place the glass container in a cool and dark place. Most people put it in the garage, basement or closet. You want the herbs to be covered and not exposed to light, as well as cool and dry. Let this sit for six weeks and you can then decant some into a smaller container and begin to use it. Apply it to injuries after the initial swelling has gone done. Or you can purchase pre-made bottles from various suppliers.

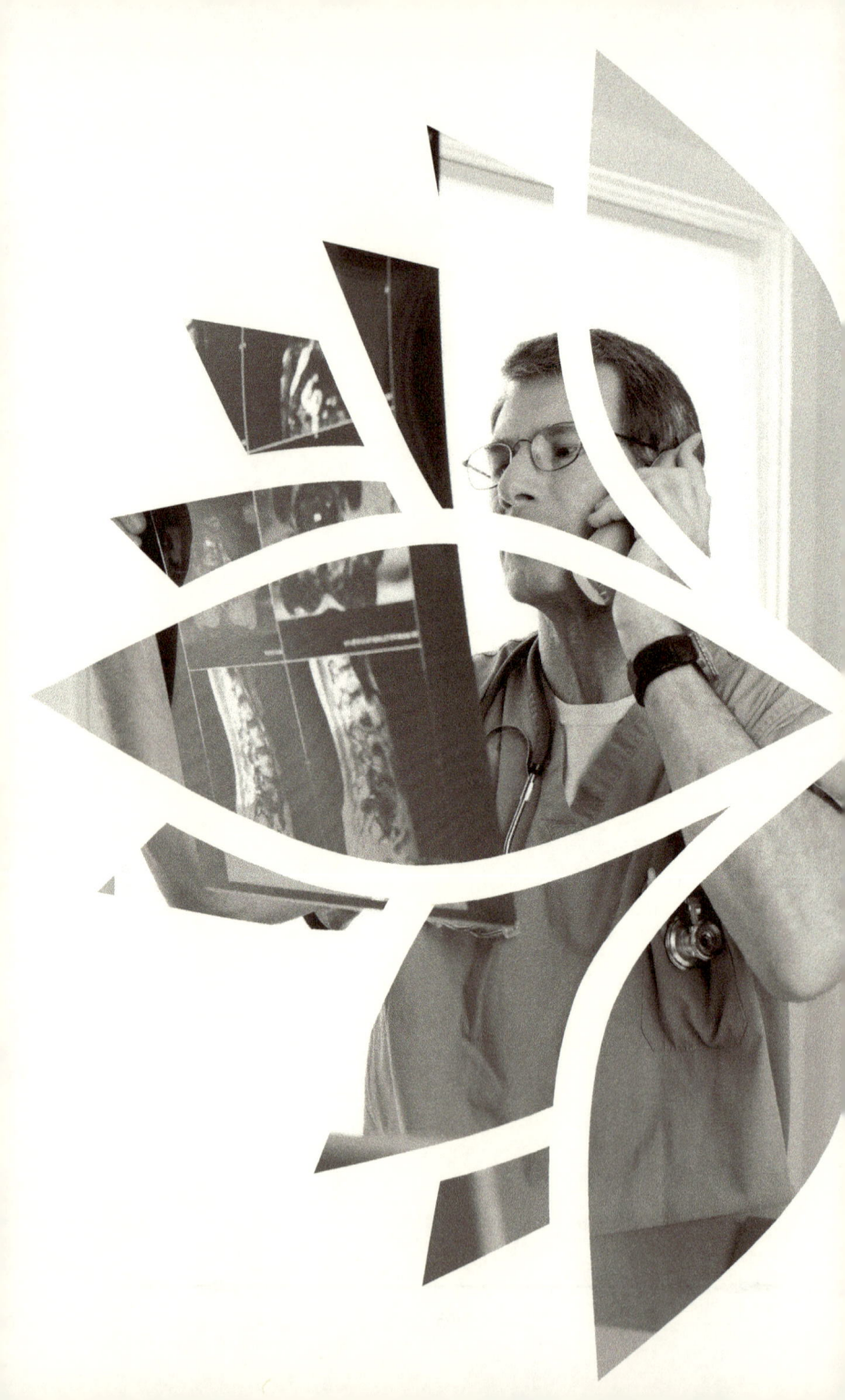

CHAPTER 13

WHEN NATURAL THERAPY ISN'T ENOUGH

Although I am a practitioner of traditional and so-called alternative medicine and health practices, I also believe in the right use of modern scientific medicines and procedures. By "right use," I mean when the big guns are used in the right situation and at the right time.

For acute issues that arise from virus, some infections, bruises, strains, inflammation, pain and the like, I advocate for taking a natural route that is easy on the body and gentle in action and that allows natural therapies time to work before escalating to chemical drugs and invasive procedures.

On the other hand, if you are in a car accident, have a headache that lasts a week and won't go away, can't stop convulsing or have other such serious medical issues, it is well-advised to seek a more scientific medical approach. There is nothing wrong with getting X-rays, MRIs and ultrasounds in addition to taking some form of anti-inflammatory or steroidal when the issue requires it.

THE EVERYDAY ACHES

Often, natural methods can handle the day-to-day aches, pains, allergies and issues that modern scientific medicine cannot. If you have chronic low back pain, medical experts agree that they are unable to eradicate it in most patients. Acupuncture, however, was ranked by the World Health Organization (WHO) as the most successful therapy for low back pain. (It was second only to placebo. While acupuncture is more powerful than Class 2 painkillers for relieving low back pain, the power of the mind is more powerful than acupuncture. Believe it.)

I have been suffering chronic migraine headaches and musculoskeletal pain nearly my entire life. And when it comes to low back pain, hip pain and groin pain, I am the king of pain. At about the age of 10, the ball joint of my hip joint slipped moderately off its growth plate. The technical term is slipped capital femoral epiphysis (SCFE; pronounced skiffy).

The hip joint is known as a ball and socket, where the ball (or femoral head, round top of the thigh bone) fits nicely into the socket (cupped shape in hip opening) and motion is smooth. The growth plate is the part of the tissue that is still growing in children; and when the femoral head slips off

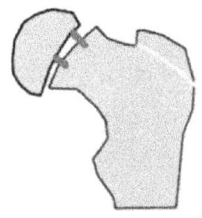 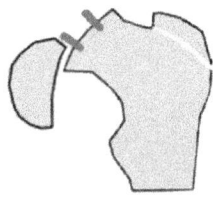

Mild	Moderate	Severe
0–1/3	1/3–2/3	2/3–complete

Change in apposition, AP projection

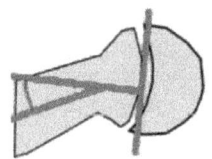 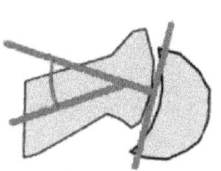 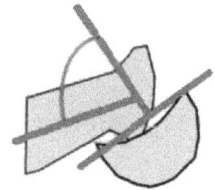

Mild	Moderate	Severe
0–30°	30–60°	60–90°

Slip angle, true lateral projection

the growth plate, the thigh bone develops into an abnormal shape. My own joint today looks more like a letter C than the proper lollipop shape.

It is not uncommon for youngsters to experience this problem. When a child or teen complains of chronic hip tightness or hip pain, has difficulty walking, one foot points inward or outward, limps and so on, he should be taken in for an X-ray. This can show the SCFE right away and two pins can be set surgically so that the issue is fixed as best it can be.

PROLONGED PROBLEMS

While I experienced all the symptoms, I never had an X-ray. I guess I spent so much time seeing specialists for my chronic migraines and shoulder and arm pain, that the hip seemed less severe. Plus, I could always explain away the symptoms as being something else.

It wasn't until I was 43 that my hip pain went from chronic to acute and jumped on a pain scale from a 4 to a 9.5.

I tried additional physical therapy, and it failed me – too much pain, more after therapy than before.

Acupuncture no longer worked. Topical pain relieving gels and creams had only nominal results anymore. It was time for the big guns: X-ray and MRI. The results showed that I now had bone-on-bone osteoarthritis as a result of slipped capitol femoral epiphysis that happened when I was about 10 years old. My orthopedists were amazed that I was able to live this long without the need for steroidal injections, strong anti-inflammatory and analgesic medications.

A TIME AND A PLACE

As I mentioned, there is a time and a place for natural and holistic medicine and a time for modern scientific medicine and invasive intervention. For me, I was able to successfully live with arthritis induced by SCFE for over 30 years by using the natural pain-relief methods I reveal in the bonus report you got with this book. It tells my story in detail, and all of the natural methods I used for staving off surgery and toxic medications for decades.

I implemented a regime of topical pain-relieving creams and gels from modern American companies and traditional Chinese medicine. I tried a wide range of therapies, including Sombra®, dimethyl sulfoxide (DMSO), and Po Sum On and Wong Luk oils. They worked great at improving blood flow, increasing range of motion, reducing stiffness and keeping me active.

For inflammation, I relied on turmeric in my diet, as well as other thermogenic spices like garlic, cloves, ginger and onion. I took capsules of butcher's broom and white willow bark daily. I reduced my intake of packaged and prepared foods, along with cutting back on sugar and alcohol. All of those promote inflammation and, thus, pain.

I also set for myself a firm sleep/wake cycle so my body could rest and repair. I engaged in mind/body practices like yoga, qigong and meditation to relax my nervous system and thereby induce the so-called relaxation response, which is just amazing at reducing pain.

When I needed outside help for the worst of times, I went to massage therapy, chiropractic, acupuncture and other such practitioners to give me a boost. These helped me relieve enough pain that I could continue with my routine.

I find that I have now moved from the natural to the scientific realm in relation to my condition. I have osteoarthritis, but not the kind that can be reversed without surgery because the root cause of it is not daily activities or age, but the SCFE. So I am at a place where for 35 years I could use natural remedies and practices to reduce inflammation and pain and enjoy my life, and now I need the "big guns."

So I have had to get total hip replacement surgery. I don't like drugs or surgery, but I am sure glad a surgery exists that can restore my hip joint to a place it has not been since I was a child. Without it, I fear I could not again enjoy life.

Wellness is a continuum that starts at prevention, proceeds to natural remedies then to chemical help and finally to surgery. There is a time and a place for them all. Again, I advocate implementing the natural at the early stages and the allopathic modern medical approaches at more serious times. Problems arise when people think acupuncture can cure cancer or surgery is needed to fix low back pain. Everything in its time and place is the best policy.

Even with growth defects, you can be sure that the natural approaches can be most effective. They have been for me, in my life of recurring pain. But when the time comes that they are no longer as effective, it is time to accept stronger, more invasive or chemically toxic therapies. They are most effective when used at the right time along the pain and injury continuum.

Now that my surgery was successfully completed, I again applied my natural and traditional methods to rehabilitate myself, strengthen my body, and bring new life back into the flow.

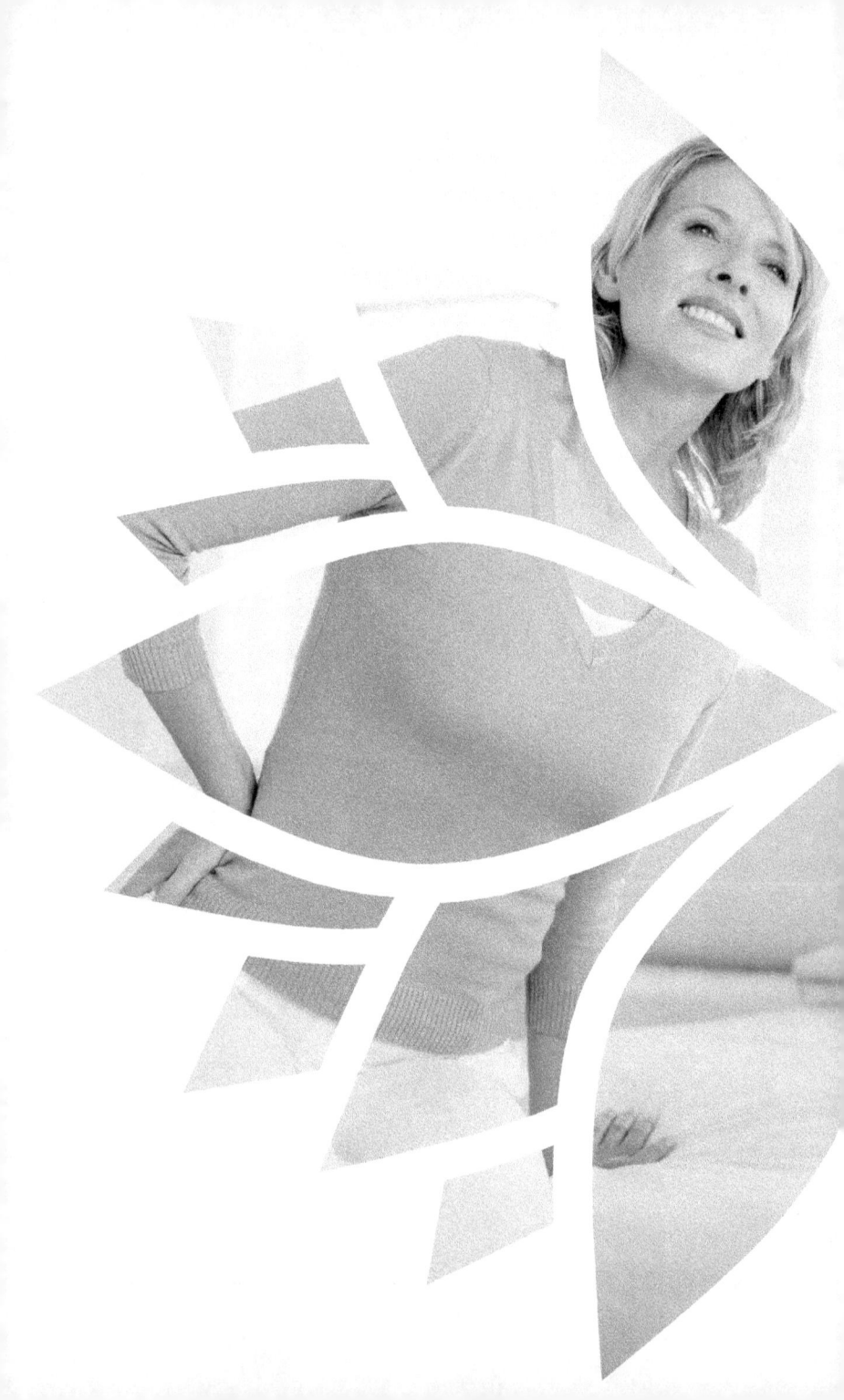

CHAPTER 14

WHEN PAIN WON'T GO AWAY, IT MAY BE TENSION MYOSITIS SYNDROME

*D*o you experience chronic or intermittent low back pain, along with a series of different types of ailments? Have you tried to manage that pain and reduce those symptoms with various medications and treatment modalities to no avail? They all may have a single root cause in common; and unless that root is corrected or addressed, the adverse health symptoms will continue. If you have tried everything without any relief, then Tension Myositis Syndrome (TMS) may be the culprit.

TMS DEFINED

Tension Myositis Syndrome (TMS) is a relatively unknown and somewhat recent health diagnostic category. It was first theorized in the 1970s by John Sarno, MD, as being a psychosomatic or mind-body disorder: a musculoskeletal neurological disorder created by the mind and emotions that changes one's physiology and causes pain and other symptoms.

Essentially, it is believed that stress and repressed emotions like anger and anxiety are the root cause of chronic back pain and a host of other disorders (discussed below). The theory of TMS, though not widely accepted in mainstream medicine yet, contends that repressed emotional triggers affect the nervous system which, in turn, slows blood flow to muscles, nerves and connective tissue. It basically causes a reaction or process that starves the body of oxygen, causing pain. This pain then becomes the location of focus and concern, alleviating the need (superficially) for dealing with the stress, anxiety and other emotional issues at hand. TMS case studies show that as the emotional components are dealt with successfully, the physical ailments that were heretofore intractable disappear almost instantly.

TMS SYMPTOMS

While pain in general (low back pain in particular) seems to be the most common symptom of TMS, it is not the only one. Generalized stiffness and numbness and tingling in the body or limbs are also associated with the syndrome. Flare-ups from painful to severe come and go at different times, showing the correlation of symptoms to (perhaps) the emotional state of the individual at any given time.

Many who experience the problems of chronic pain, tension headache, fibromyalgia, irritable bowel syndrome (IBS), constipation, arm pain, temporal mandibular joint dysfunction (TMJD) and tinnitus (ringing in the ears) have had difficulty finding relief or cure from mainstream approaches. They may have the basis or root of their symptoms in TMS.

TMS EQUIVALENCE

As a mind-body practitioner myself, and as someone who has suffered debilitating headaches and musculoskeletal pain for most of my life, I have always thought the psychosomatic (mind-body) connection plays a central role in our daily state of health. What I find intriguing about TMS is its theory of equivalence; it offers a connection not generally made in the mainstream or alternative health communities. Here are four short passages from Sarno's book, *Healing Back Pain*, that are interesting, informative and thought-provoking:

- *"TMS is equivalent to peptic ulcer, spastic colitis, constipation, tension headache, migraine headache, cardiac palpitations, eczema, allergic rhinitis (hay fever), prostatitis (often), ringing in the ears (often) and dizziness (often)."*
- *"I believe these disorders are interchangeable and equivalent of each other because many of them are found to occur historically in patients with TMS, sometimes at the same time, but often in tandem."*
- *"Equivalence is also suggested by the fact that patients often report resolution of one of these disorders when the TMS*

pain goes away. This happens most commonly with hay fever. I teach patients that all the conditions on the list serve the same purpose psychologically."

- *"Experience with TMS and these related conditions suggests that there may be a common denominator, anxiety perhaps, that can bring on any of these disorders. In that case, some other emotion, anger for example, may be the primary one that may in turn induce anxiety, which then brings on the symptom."*

TMS TREATMENT

Patients bring their medical history when consulting with a TMS physician. This information generally includes written physician reports, lab results and diagnostic imaging studies. After receiving a diagnosis of TMS, treatment begins.

The first step in treating TMS requires patient education. Physicians generally provide audio and written materials or recommend lectures. Education teaches the patient various aspects of the condition and reassures them that physical symptoms do not occur because of typical disease processes, physical injury or re-injury.

Another treatment modality physicians may use for treating TMS involves keeping a daily journal and writing about circumstances that might have created repressed emotional stress. David Schechter, MD, recommends that when patients begin writing, they should consider whether they relate to certain key areas that often contribute to repressed feelings:

- Abuse, abandonment or neglect during childhood.
- Conscientiousness or perfectionism related to acceptance.
- Current life stressors.
- Aging or mortality.
- Situations wherein patients feel but repress negative emotions.

After identifying a list of possible contributing factors, TMS physicians require that patients formulate an essay for each of the problem areas. Longer essays provide patients with the opportunity of exploring the issue in greater detail. Schechter developed a 30-day program called *The MindBody Workbook*, which assists patients with documenting events that trigger negative emotions. The journal helps patients correlate the emotion with the physical symptoms of TMS. Over time, patients learn to use emotional expression rather than repression.

Part of TMS treatment also requires that patients live as if symptom-free. If physicians find no physical reason for chronic pain, Schechter advises that patients stop using conventional treatment methods for pain control. He believes these methods serve only to mentally reinforce a physical condition that does not exist. Patients must also resume normal physical activities when there is no physical evidence for pain.

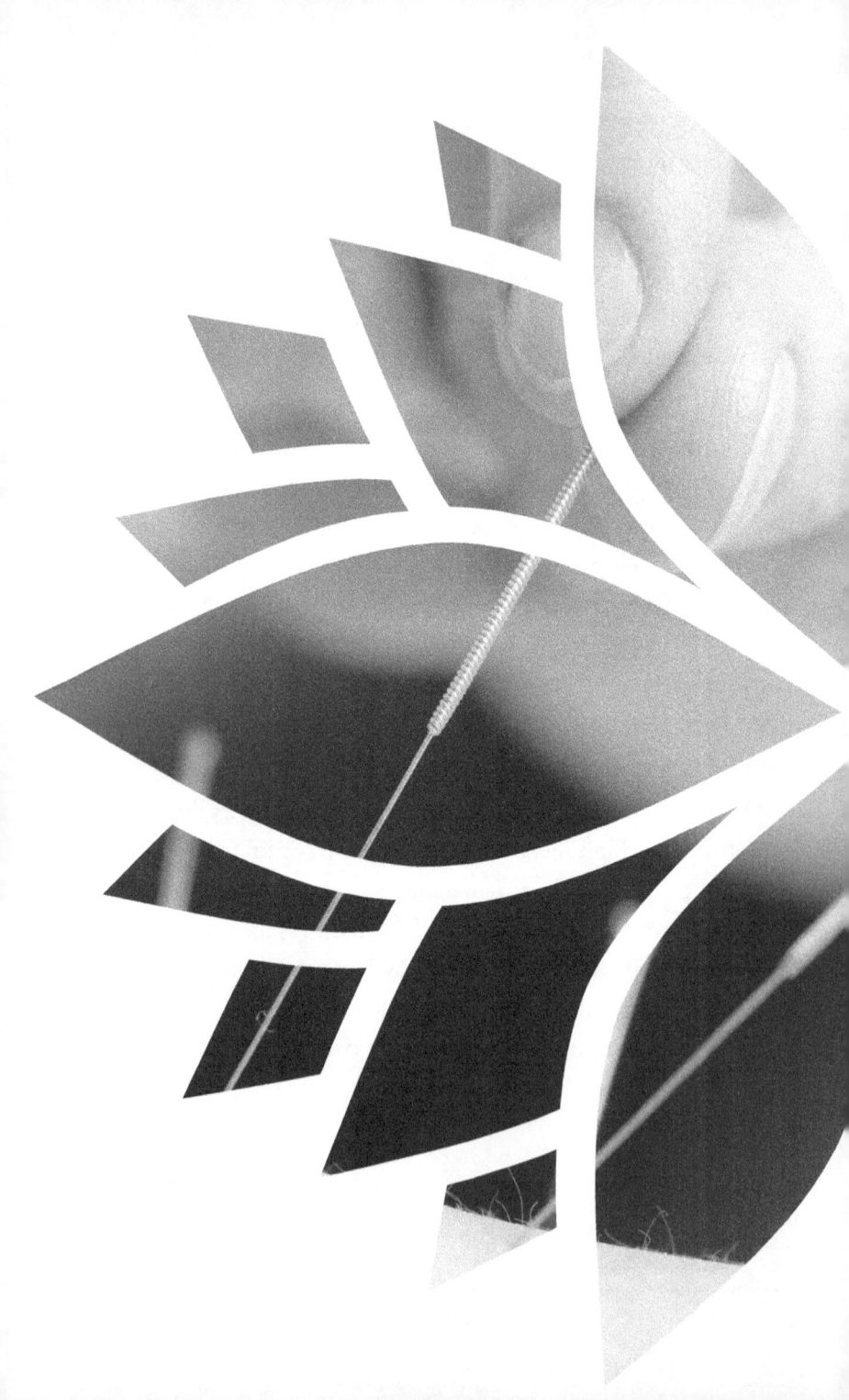

CHAPTER 15

THE NEWEST – AND OLDEST – IN ALTERNATIVE ANTI-PAIN THERAPIES

ACUPUNCTURE OFFERS BETTER PAIN RELIEF

Although many conventional doctors doubt the effectiveness of acupuncture, this venerated medical technique produces profound benefits. Research at Duke University, for example, shows that acupuncture sessions can lead to significant pain relief. And the wonderful results of acupuncture are much more desirable than what you get from pain relief drugs and their troubling side effects.

ACUPUNCTURE BENEFITS

For thousands of years, the Chinese have been using a unique method of health maintenance called acupuncture. Today, acupuncture is a household word and part of America's out-of-pocket healthcare toolbox. But this ancient needle-and-channel therapy remains an outlier when it comes to acceptance in the mainstream medical establishment. However, a pair of studies coming out of Duke University that shed positive light on the benefits of acupuncture over drugs for pain relief represents an important step toward giving acupuncture more Western credibility.

In one report, researchers at Duke performed a meta-analysis of 31 clinical studies involving some 4,000 patients on the effects of acupuncture for headache relief compared to treatment with medication. Their findings: *"Acupuncture is more effective than medication in reducing the severity and frequency of chronic headaches."*

When comparing the data, the researchers found that 62% of those given acupuncture for headaches reported pain relief. Only 45% of those taking medication for their head pain reported relief. Two important points to take note of: The studies were conducted on people suffering various types of headaches (tension, migraine, etc.) and proper acupuncture point prescription was essential.

DISTURBING DRUGS

As a former chronic headache sufferer myself, the thing I find most disturbing and unreliable about conventional treatment is the fact that each time you seek pain relief for a varying kind of headache, you are prescribed almost the identical medication.

Consider the fact that most over-the-counter headache medications are basically the same formula even though you may be taking them for pain with different causes. So even though the symptoms and mechanisms leading to migraines differ from those causing sinus, tension, cluster and other types of headaches, Western doctors don't differentiate in their treatments. This is true despite the fact that treating them all in the same way is neither useful nor effective.

ACCURATE ACUPUNCTURE

Acupuncture stimulates different points in the body that fall along energy lines called meridians. Depending on the location of the headache (top of head, side of head) and the type of symptoms associated with the pain (throbbing, burning, sweating), the practitioner alters the points being stimulated by the acupuncture needles. Consequently, the acupuncture is used differently for different headache types and locations. It is, therefore, more specific. However, the theory on which the therapy is based remains unchanged: Where there is blockage of energy in the body, there is pain. Release the blockage; diminish the pain.

And while several studies seem to show that sham acupuncture (using non-specific points) offers some relief, the Duke study found that the greatest relief of pain is gained from using correct needle technique administered to the correct acupoints.

"One of the barriers to treatment with acupuncture," says Dr. Tong Joo Gan, the study lead, *"is getting people to understand that while needles are used, it is not a painful experience. It is a method for releasing your body's own natural painkillers."* Gan is correct. In fact, the needles used in acupuncture are so thin that they can be tied into a knot with two fingers. Those who fear the pain associated with the hypodermic needles used in medical shots are reassured to know that 20 acupuncture needles can fit into the opening of the standard medical needle. Acupuncture needles are so thin, in fact, that you can insert one of these needles into an inflated balloon and the balloon does not pop.

MORE THAN ONE SESSION

Acupuncture is not a one-off treatment for headaches, though. Since the theory of its use is based on removing imbalances in the body to allow free flow of energy, fluids and nerve signals, it often takes several visits to feel the results. Ten treatments in a row are often considered "one course of treatment," with more than one course being necessary for chronic conditions.

In another analysis of 15 studies, Duke University Medical Center anesthesiologists found that when acupuncture is administered both before and during surgery, there is a significant reduction in the pain experienced by patients and less postsurgical opioids (potent pain killers) needed to control pain.

Presenting his findings at the annual scientific conference of the American Society for Anesthesiology in San Francisco, Gan stated, *"While the amount of opioids needed for patients who received acupuncture was much lower than those who did not have acupuncture, the most important outcome for the patient is the reduction of the side effects associated with opioids. These side effects can negatively impact a patient's recovery from surgery and lengthen the time spent in the hospital."*

The meta-analysis showed that the risk of developing the side effects of opioids after surgery was significantly lower in those patients who were administered acupuncture before and during surgery, compared with the control group. Specifically, acupuncture patients experienced *"1.5 times lower rates of nausea; 1.3 times fewer incidences of severe itching; 1.6 times fewer reports of dizziness and 3.5 times fewer cases of urinary retention."*

This is good news for the acupuncture community, and especially for those who seek more holistic and less toxic methods for pain relief. Acupuncture has been perfected over the past 5,000 years in China, the most populated country in the world. Allopathic medicine, in comparison, is still in its infancy. Yet, in the United States, where modern drugs rule the roost, acupuncture is still seen as hokey, and acupuncturists are not accepted as "doctors" by the American Medical Association (AMA).

Well, we live in a new age now, and studies like these done by reputable universities based on clinical data do much to show the mainstream establishment that ancient remedies and health practices are as valid today as ever. In the case of pain control, these types of holistic therapies are more powerful and less toxic than the usual drugs.

STEP INTO THE DOORWAY TO PAIN RELIEF

Sudden stiffness and pain can strike any time, any place, anywhere on the body. But you don't have to suffer without fighting back. The key to quick pain relief: Release the tightness and stretch painful muscles to bring fresh blood to the area and restore range of motion. All you need is a doorway to anchor a few simple stretches.

COMMON PAIN

Among the most common pain spots on the body are the chest, shoulders and upper back. You know this pain well and you see others experiencing it, too. It seems like when one of these areas gets tight, the others follow suit.

Pain can arrive in the form of nagging shoulder pain, neck pain, pain behind the shoulder blades, pain in the chest and, soon, headaches. Anti-inflammatories or analgesics are OK in a pinch. Massage and chiropractic are good, too. The best bet, however, is to release the stiffness before it gets worse and pain sets in.

Neck, chest and shoulder stiffness usually comes from poor posture and stress. Often people are hunched over their desks on a computer all day and this elongates the muscles in the shoulder while compressing the muscles in the chest. When your muscles are all jammed up, they hurt. No worries: When you're in a jam, use the jamb to release the pain.

The door jamb, that is.

FEEL YOUR PAIN

The first thing to do when experiencing shoulder, chest and upper back stiffness or pain is to try and feel it. This lets you better understand the tightness and where it originates.

If your neck hurts, but not your shoulders, for example, then the pain may be from sleeping in an uncomfortable position. If your shoulders hurt, it could be from sleeping with your arm above your head or from stress. Additionally, the shoulders could be tightening because of shortened chest muscles, or pecs. These get short or contracted when the arms are held close in front of the body for extended periods of time when typing, writing, driving or reading. Postural and behavioral changes go a long way to prevent the tightness and pain from returning.

When the chest muscles tighten, they cause your shoulders to round forward. This gives you what personal trainers often call "turtle back." This just means your upper back and shoulders are hunched forward, which causes pain as they keep your chest muscles in a constant state of tightness or contraction and your shoulders in an extended position. This makes your shoulders contract in an effort to pull them back to a normal position. The prolonged contraction leads to trigger points, those nasty knots you feel in your shoulders. They are painful.

PAINFUL DILEMMA

When experiencing chronic shoulder, chest, and upper back pain, many grab for NSAIDs (nonsteroidal anti-inflammatory drugs), hot compresses and showers, chiropractic adjustments and acupuncture. Others opt for massage and some even go so far as to get physical therapy. The best advice I can give on any pain issue is to start low-tech and try the least invasive approach first. Often times, the simplest thing is the fastest solution.

In this case, it's stretching in a doorway. Here are five ways you can do it:

DOORWAY STRETCH ONE:

- Stand with feet parallel and just behind the doorway.
- Place your right forearm against the doorway frame. Make sure your arm is held at a 90-degree angle with palm flat against the jamb.
- Step forward with your right foot through to the other side of the doorway. Do not move your arm. You should feel a nice stretch across your right pectoral (chest) muscle. Hold for 20 seconds.
- If it is too painful to hold this position, take a shorter step forward.
- If you do not feel the stretch, then turn your torso toward the left while keeping everything else in place.
- After 20 seconds, return to the starting position by stepping back with your right foot.
- Repeat on the left side.

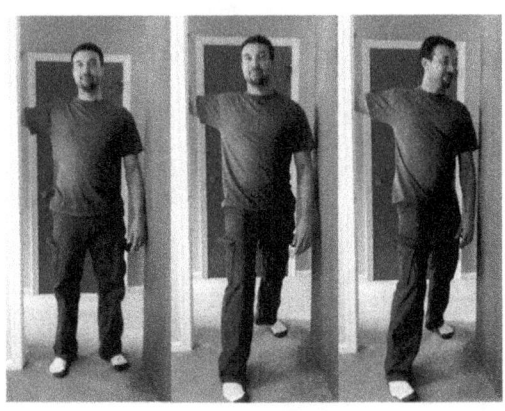

DOORWAY STRETCH TWO:

- Stand with feet parallel and just behind the doorway.
- Place your right forearm against the doorway frame. Make sure your arm is held at a 120-degree angle with palm flat against the jamb.
- Step forward with your right foot through to the other side of the doorway. Do not move your arm. You should feel a nice stretch across your right pectoral (chest) muscle. Hold for 20 seconds.
- If it is too painful to hold this position, take a shorter step forward.
- If you do not feel the stretch, then turn your torso toward the left while keeping everything else in place.
- After 20 seconds, return to the starting position by stepping back with your right foot.
- Repeat on the left side.

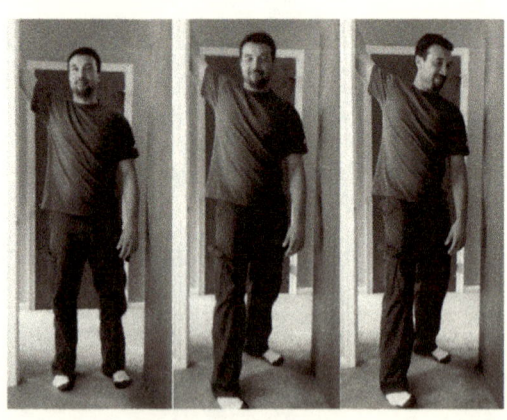

DOORWAY STRETCH THREE:

- Stand with feet parallel and just behind the doorway. Or, if you are too tall to allow a full arm extension toward the top of the doorway, kneel behind the doorway.
- Place your right forearm against the inside of the doorway frame.
- Slowly slide your arm up along the inside of the doorway frame. You should feel a nice stretch across your right pectoral (chest) muscle and around your shoulders and rotators.
- If you do not feel the stretch, lean slightly forward and that should do the trick.
- Hold for 20 seconds then return to the starting position by slowly sliding your arm back down the frame.
- Repeat on the left side.

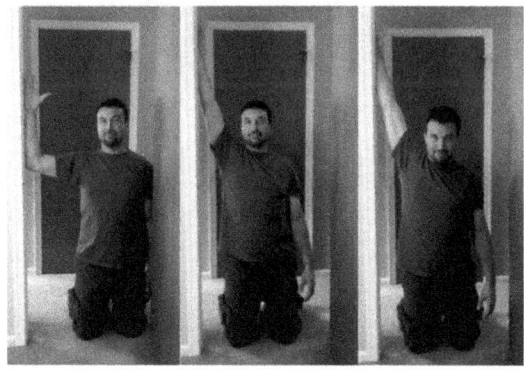

DOORWAY STRETCH FOUR:

- Stand with feet parallel and just behind the doorway.
- Place the palms of both hands flat on the back of the jamb, forearms held parallel to the floor.
- Slowly allow your upper body to lean forward and hold for 20 seconds. You should feel a stretch across your chest, along your ribs and/or between your shoulder blades.
- After 20 seconds, return to the starting position. This is the warm-up for the next stretch.

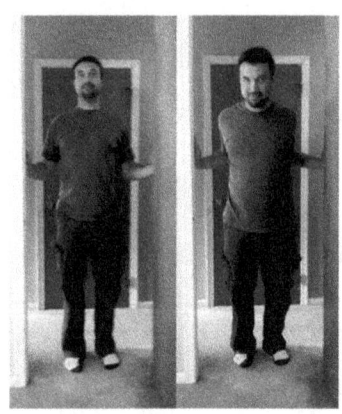

DOORWAY STRETCH FIVE:

- Stand with feet parallel and just behind the doorway.
- Place your forearms flat along the back of the jamb, triceps held parallel to the floor.
- Slowly allow your upper body to lean forward and hold for 20 seconds. You should feel a stretch across your chest, along your ribs and/or between your shoulder blades.
- After 20 seconds, return to the starting position.

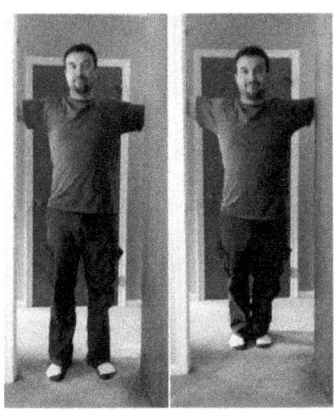

There are many ways a door jamb can be used to stretch the upper and lower parts of your body. These are just a few examples to get you started. The secret to the benefits of these doorway stretches is doing them slow and steady.

Correcting your posture and moving every hour away from your desk also helps prevent the chest, shoulders and upper back from tightening. But if they do, these stretches are a doorway to pain relief.

ALIGN BODY, MIND AND GRAVITY TO BANISH PAIN

There are two factors that are unavoidable and wreak havoc on our bodies: stress and gravity. Gravity, of course, is not something we can change; but we can manage our lives to account for it. Stress is something that comes in physical, mental and emotional forms and also needs to be managed. Over time, stress changes our musculature and our physical form. And when the force of gravity encounters those rounded shoulders and hunched backs caused by stress, pain and discomfort are hard to avoid.

WORKING THE BODY

I'm a big fan of bodywork, especially when combined with mind/body practices. Having suffered chronic and debilitating body pain for most of my life, I make it a point to try as many bodywork methods as I can, both old and new. I even made the study of Tui-Na (from China), Thai yoga massage and hilot (from the Philippines) part of my formal education training. I also use muscle-energy technique, neuromuscular technique, positional release and many others to help myself and my clients.

There is a bodywork method developed in the 1930s that is less popular today, but should be revisited by pain sufferers. Originally known as "structural integration," this method was developed by a woman named Ida Rolf. Now known as Rolfing®, this was among the first Western bodywork methods to address pain through posture and the quality of fascia (connective tissue) in relationship to the Earth's gravitational pull.

PAIN THEORY

What makes Rolfing® special? Well, by the age of 25, Rolf had earned a PhD in biochemistry from the College of Physicians and Surgeons at Columbia University, then traveled to Geneva to study homeopathic medicine. She derived a theory about pain and discomfort that led her to look at the body's connective tissue, or fascia.

Fascia is the web-like tissue that encapsulates individual muscles, groups of muscles, blood vessels and nerves. Characteristically, fascia is designed to protect parts of the body but also to allow certain internal structures (like muscles) to slide or glide over others.

Connective tissue protects, but sometimes it is too protective. In many instances, for example, an injury causes more fascia to be made to shield the damaged area. When this new growth overcompensates, and when the original injury is healed, the fascia remains like a fortress, not allowing free range of motion. But there doesn't have to be an injury to make this happen.

USE IT OR LOSE IT

When you don't use your limbs in all the directions in which they are designed to be manipulated (think of the ball-and-socket nature of your shoulders), the fascia eventually adheres or sticks together.

In normal circumstances, the fascia should allow the musculature of the shoulder, neck and back to slide. But because of limited use of the arms by most people (by holding them fixed in place while typing, etc.), the fascia grows sticky and prevents the natural slide. This causes range of motion issues, stiffness, soreness and pain. This also happens with our hips and lower backs from prolonged sitting and a lack of walking and other exercise.

While this understanding is now common knowledge, back in the 1930s it was revolutionary in the West to think of pain in these terms. But Rolf had a eureka moment and made this argument: Every person has an optimal alignment of the body, an optimal range of motion for his body type, and, thus, an easier way for the body to interact with gravity. When this natural and optimal relationship is distorted with stressful actions, thoughts and behaviors and unnatural use of the body, the connective tissue adheres and causes internal stress and discomfort. It changes the way the body stands, sits, rests and lies. It causes pain. And this happens in relationship to the way gravity works to hold us down and pulls on us.

GRAVITY'S TOLL

When we are hunched, tilted or crooked, gravity pulls us further out of shape.

Here is a description from the Rolfing® website that says it better than I can: "Preventing discomfort is one of the objectives of Rolfing®. By engaging with the self and the earth's gravity and establishing the optimal individual alignment, the client has a greater capacity to function to the best of his or her individual ability. This is in line with Dr. Rolf's belief that there is something of an inherent best individual alignment, realized through Rolfing®."

Rolfers (Rolfing® practitioners) seek to correct the misalignment of the body during 10 sessions that realign the connective tissue to return it to normal function. This is done, sometimes with painful and sometimes gentle massage techniques, to eliminate or limit the body's internal stress, to return the normal range of motion and realign the body so it can relate to gravity optimally.

When Rolf said, "fascia is the organ of form," she was spot on. And when she suggested that, "deliberate, accurate and targeted movement of this tissue" could lead to instant relief of physical pain and increase well-being and quality of life, she began a bodywork revolution that continues to this day. In my estimation, the late Rolf was one of the originators of Western-based mind/body medicine, taking into consideration the combined role of stress, mind, body and gravity in health and well-being.

And while Rolfing® is no longer called "structural integration," that is its aim. All of you who have poor posture, visit chiropractors and massage therapists, and are looking for relief for chronic body pain should give Rolfing® a try. Better yet, don't try it, commit to a 10-session program and see how it can make you feel freer and happier.

For more information on Rolfing® and to find a practitioner visit www.rolfing.org

AWARENESS AND PAIN RELIEF THROUGH "OPPOSITE" MOVEMENT

In the not-too-distant past, the term "psychosomatic" was a bad word.

Many healthcare practitioners did not yet understand it, and people with unexplainable illnesses and pain were told (and came to believe) that their problems were all "in their minds." Since the 1990s, however, research proves what the ancients knew: The mind and body are one. Both relate to and can affect each other in positive and negative ways. With this knowledge, the stigma of psychosomatic has been lifted, and mind/body practices are helping millions of Americans.

Although in China and India mind/body practices abound and were developed thousands of years ago, they are relatively new in the West. Practices like yoga, meditation, tai chi and qigong are known to almost everyone these days (even if relatively few people engage in these activities).

These methods teach one to quiet the mind, coordinate the breath and sync bodily movements or hold particular postures.

All of this is designed to achieve an inner harmony between mind and body, regulate the nervous system and quiet the mind to allow the body to heal itself.

While the Asian systems of mind/body are well-known, there is a method developed in the West that is less familiar but which I find extremely beneficial. Although I am not a certified practitioner of this method, I have been guided through it and refer back to it as needed. It is called the Feldenkrais Method®.

SIMPLE CONCEPT

The Feldenkrais Method® is named after its founder, Moshé Feldenkrais. The method is quite simple in concept. It uses movement in directions often opposite to what you are used to in order to retrain the body to improve movement and coordination.

It's supposed to help make the connection between thoughts and feelings and how they manifest in the body as cramps, tight muscles, muscle imbalances, impingements and pain.

Feldenkrais' principles can be applied in every orientation, direction, pattern and activity that we engage in.

1. **Good posture** is the ability to move in any direction without hesitation or preparation.
2. **Clear skeletal support:** The bones below move to support the bones above.
3. **Evenly distributed muscular effort/tone** (proportional work: The big muscles do the big work, small muscles small work).
4. Every movement is generated through an **equal and opposite** force delivered to/received from the ground.
5. **Force must travel up and through** the skeleton (longitudinally), not across it. Avoid shearing forces.
6. **Head and eyes are free** in the activity.
7. **Breathing is free** in the activity.
8. **Reversibility:** The ability to organize for the action and its suspension or reversal at any moment. (Source: bodyofknowledge.me)

While the Asian mind/body systems popular in the West today have specialized meditative or internal energy components, Feldenkrais is a bit different. It is a therapy that allows practitioners to help clients improve general awareness of the body and themselves. This is discovered through a practice of observing and examining the specific thought-to-movement relationships that, when negative, often manifest as limited range of motion, stiffness and physical pain. Discovering these relationships helps begin the process of reducing pain and stiffness while expanding range of motion.

Those who experience the effects of the Feldenkrais Method® are fond of saying: "Learning to move with less effort makes daily life easier." And this is true when the body's natural range of motion is re-set, causing muscle imbalance, spasms and pains that were caused by an imbalanced body to decrease and disappear over time. This allows more enjoyment of life. When you can do simple activities like tying shoes, bending over or making a cup of tea, then your everyday life can be immensely joyful and healing – especially if you have suffered for years.

Again, it is through guided movement practices that the Feldenkrais Method® teaches you to improve your capabilities to function in daily life. These movements help coordinate and connect mind and body, not for meditation or energy building, but for a joyful life through improved abilities to carry out the activities of daily living.

TWO PHASES

There are two methods or phases to learning the Feldenkrais Method® termed "Awareness Through Movement" and "Functional Integration." The first phase is learned in a class setting where participants are verbally guided through different movement sequences for 30-to-60 minutes. During this time, they are encouraged to explore the content and the methods they employ when they think, sense, move and imagine during their ordinary functional movements in daily life.

This series of guided movements is easy to learn and is performed slowly, yet it builds over time into more complex movements that increase range of motion through release of tension and blockages in the body.

Each class session is structured around a specific body movement function wherein a series of movements is taught to help relearn and retrain awkward body movement and rebalance the mind. In other words, "Awareness Through Movement" aims to "make one aware of his/her habitual neuromuscular patterns and rigidities and to expand options for new ways of moving while increasing sensitivity and improving efficiency."

FUNCTIONAL INTEGRATION

Functional Integration sessions are hands-on methods wherein the Feldenkrais Method® practitioner works like a physical therapist or body worker to stretch shortened muscles. Unlike the sometimes harsh pressing and rubbing of deep-tissue massage, Functional Integration techniques are gentle and noninvasive. They are described by practitioners as being a form of "tactile, kinesthetic communication."

Through the session, a practitioner is able to feel and sense what is going on in the client's body and tell him how to better organize the body through guided movement and how to move in more expanded functional motor patterns.

While not steeped in altered states of consciousness and internal energy like its Asian counterparts, the Feldenkrais Method® is no less effective at aligning the body and improving its functions through an intimate mind/body awareness.

I found this method to be helpful for me when other methods failed to reach a source for muscular imbalances that lead to limited range of motion and pain in my own body. It connected my imbalances with mental processes. Working on the mind and the body concurrently and understanding their connection are powerful tools to improving well-being and quality of life. For more information on the Feldenkrais Method®, visit www.feldenkrais.com.

BANISH PAIN AND STIFFNESS WITH THE MUSCLE ENERGY TECHNIQUE

One of the most debilitating and emotionally frustrating ailments is limited range of motion. That occurs when the hands, arms, hips and legs are supposed to move freely within a "normal" range and area, but they can't. They are held captive by pain, muscle spasms, trigger points, constricted tendons and inflamed joints.

When this continues over time and becomes chronic, you have to alter your daily activities. And this doesn't merely limit your ability to play a sport or go for a long walk, but restricts your capacity for opening cabinets and reaching for things on shelves. This limited range of motion causes pain, emotional turmoil and loss of zest for life. But an old technique, nearly lost in today's healthcare practices, can help enormously.

THE LOST ART

Back in the day, osteopathic medicine was cool. It was aligned with naturalistic medicine and preventive care. It treated the external body through bodywork methods and internally with diet and medicines. It was holistic. My father is a retired doctor of osteopathy (DO); the old guard (that included him) has been replaced by a new guard. During their education, they take an elective in the bodywork method of spinal manipulation and muscle energy technique, but they soon forget what they've learned.

When I press my colleagues in this field on why they no longer (or ever) offered this modality to patients, they often say it takes too much time, they have too many patients to see and that people want drugs – not therapy. I disagree. This is not the case for all DOs, so ask yours (if you have one) about the little- known method known as Muscle Energy Technique, or MET.

Depending on which history you ascribe to, osteopathic medicine was the first Western mainstream medical system in the United States to employ somatic manipulative diagnosis and treatment. That is, it palpated (touched) the body to assess muscle tension and imbalances, to maneuver the limbs to assess range of motion and to correct spinal misalignment with manipulation techniques and fixed muscle and joint dysfunction with stretching and controlled force.

Legend has it that the first osteopath learned spinal manipulation from a Chinese doctor working on the railroads. This makes sense: Traditional Chinese medicine (TCM) has hundreds of such techniques in its Tui Na curriculum. And chiropractic, it is said, is a breakaway system from osteopathic medicine, focusing almost exclusively on spinal health and manipulation. Sports medicine's use of a method known as proprioceptive neuromuscular facilitation (PNF) is said to be a direct descendant of osteopathic MET.

MUSCLE ENERGY TECHNIQUE DESCRIBED

MET is a method of somatic correction (joint and muscle corrective therapy) in which the patient and the doctor work together to activate the injured, shortened or stiff muscle. From precise and controlled positions, the patient is asked to use force to press his limb (held in a specific position based on diagnosis and muscles treated) against opposing force from the doctor's hands. This, in effect, re-sets the muscle tone and bone structure toward normalcy to restore normal range of motion and decrease pain.

How it works is that muscle energy is used, or energy is applied through muscle flexing, against a fixed restrictive barrier, usually the doctor's hand. The doctor places his hand on the side of the knee, for example, of a patient lying on his back with knees bent and feet flat; and he applies an amount of force that the patient must match. The force from the muscle meets the force of the barrier, and it seems as if neither the physician's hand nor the patient's knee move. Yet internally there is much happening through the isometric contraction of the patient's muscles.

HOW IT WORKS

This simple action causes the agonistic muscle to fatigue and relax, thereby allowing the antagonistic muscle to move farther along its range of motion with less restriction and pain. There are eight basic steps to the application of MET as applied to a specific treatment site:

1. A correct somatic assessment and diagnosis is made.
2. The restrictive barrier is engaged in as many planes as possible.
3. Counterforce is matched between physician and patient, with the physician setting and managing the force.
4. The patient applies isometric force in the opposite direction of the restriction (if it hurts to pull the leg in, push it out) and holds against the physician's barrier

for five to 21 seconds, depending on what the doctor thinks is necessary.

5. After the count, the patient is asked to release all force but not move the limb from its location, thus allowing the muscles to relax completely.

6. The physician moves the patient's limb to the next barrier of pain, a new position further along the range of motion that was not possible before the session.

7. Steps 3 through 6 are repeated not more than five times in one session, as this allows the greatest change in range of motion without causing inflammation or rebound pain.

8. Somatic assessment is again made to judge how much correction has taken hold and whether further sessions are required.

WHEN MET IS APPROPRIATE

Be advised that not every type of pain and range restriction is suitable to treat with MET. For best results, MET is most suited for decreased range of motion caused by muscle spasm and tightness, hypertonic and hypotonic muscles (too tight or too lax), altered joint position and decreased elasticity in ligaments and muscles. Barring serious physical traumatic injury, people suffering stiffness, pain and limited range of motion in the legs, hips, low back, pelvis, mid back, shoulders and neck have been treated. This technique has even been successful in alleviating edema and respiratory dysfunctions.

The important thing is to consult your physician and ask if he is skilled in MET. If he is not, and if your pain and range of motion are taking a toll, tell him that you are interested in learning more about it and ask for a referral to a practitioner. It is gentler and more specific than PNF and other, similar, physical therapy and sports medicine modalities. I studied several such methods and prefer to use MET with my clients. Being assessed properly is essential to determine which joint structures or muscle groups are out of balance or alignment. This can be tricky to determine if one is untrained in the somatic diagnosis method, and so finding an educated practitioner is advised.

THE POWER OF TOUCH

The power of human touch has played an important role in the history of healing. The therapeutic power of touch is evidenced in activities like the religious ceremonial laying on of hands and faith healing sessions. It's also been used in energetic healing systems like qigong and Reiki, as well as in contemporary practices like massage, acupressure and chiropractic.

With the vast increase in prescription drugs, radiation therapies and high-tech surgical procedures, the focus on — and indeed, the belief in — the healing power of touch, has all but disappeared in mainstream medicine. It is alive and well in many alternative health venues, but remains largely a fringe method of healing.

This should not be the case.

Today, our modern scientific method has time and again rediscovered what the ancients knew all along about touch. But years ago, the conventional view held that the practice of touch was a quaint subject relegated to old books and oral folklore.

Only recently has modern science awakened to the power of touch. And new technology has shown that touch is a valid therapy.

Consequently, the power of human touch has finally been proven effective by scientific studies, especially when it comes to pain relief.

REPETITIVE PROOF

Every day, when we brush up against something, are poked or bump into objects, we experience the sensation of touch. Sometimes the sensation is pleasant. Other times it is quite painful.

Generally, the type of pain you feel, the sensation of the touch event, brings to your mind an instant picture or vision of what you had contact with. When you stub your toe, along with the pain arrives an image of the table leg. Step on something shard and pointy, and along with the pain is an image of a nail or tack or splinter (depending on the specific pain sensation, and your personal experience with that type of sensation).

This happens, according to two recent studies published in the journal *Nature,* because your epidermis conveys the feelings/sensations to the central nervous system, which equates it with something from previous experience. Cells called Merkel cells, specifically, have been thought to be involved in this process, but it was not understood just what role they played. However, the recent studies published in Nature give insight into this process:

"Recordings from touch-dome afferents lacking Merkel cells demonstrate that Merkel cells confer high-frequency responses to dynamic stimuli and enable sustained firing. [T]hese findings indicate that Merkel cells actively tune mechanosensory responses to facilitate high spatio-temporal acuity."

Additionally:

"Merkel cells signal static stimuli, such as pressure, whereas sensory afferents transduce dynamic stimuli, such as moving gratings. Thus, the Merkel cell-neurite complex is a unique sensory structure composed of two different receptor cell types specialized for distinct elements of discriminative touch...

"Our data present evidence for a two-receptor-site model, in which both Merkel cells and innervating afferents act together as mechanosensors. The two-receptor system could provide this mechanoreceptor complex with a tuning mechanism to achieve highly sophisticated responses to a given mechanical stimulus."

What this shows, for the first time, is that Merkel cells actively encode basic information about pressure that's being exerted when we touch something. And they also amplify and enhance subtler sensations such as the shape of a keyboard beneath fingertips.

MECHANISM OF TOUCH

Nature has published a pair of studies on the mechanism of touch and how it acts to reduce pain sensations in those suffering conditions like postural orthostatic tachycardia syndrome (POTS). POTS causes its victims to feel intense pain whenever they are touched.

This condition results from a dysfunctional autonomic nervous system that produces symptoms akin to fibromyalgia. With POTS, even the lightest and most tender sensations can be painful events — even from touches like a feather on the skin or the wind on your skin.

This new discovery of how humans feel and process the sensation of touch is leading the scientific community to study how sensations of touch, various pressures and motions, influence the body and its experience of pain. For people who can't even feel touch and for those who experience pain when touched, research is trying to find ways to correct the dysfunction.

As the *Nature* study's co-author and associate professor at Columbia University, Ellen Lumpkin, told Pacific Standard,

"Understanding the basis of gentle touch has implications for unrelieved pain, particularly tactile allodynia (pain when touched)."

And here we are, with science finally catching up to the wisdom of the ancients in countries across the globe, rediscovering the power and validity of the power of human touch to heal.

REFERENCES:

http://www.nature.com/nature/journal/vaop/ncurrent/full/nature13251.html

http://www.nature.com/nature/journal/vaop/ncurrent/full/nature13250.html

http://www.psmag.com/navigation/health-and-behavior/mystery-human-touch-78444/

AFTERWORD

TAKE CONTROL OF YOUR PAIN

People often find it difficult to take control of their own health and well-being. They try hard and never seem to get where they want or need to be.

I want you to know that you can stop trying to change your life and start doing it.

I myself had my old beliefs changed when confronted by patients who would not do what I asked of them between visits. I would get annoyed, frustrated and sometimes angry. I spent a lot of time with them explaining the program laid out for them and teaching them how and what to do on their own as a supplement to what I could do for them in the office.

When they complained of increasing pain or lack of a speedy recovery, I started to lose my own sense of caring about their outcomes. And this was the antithesis of my reasons for being in the healing vocation.

At first, I felt that people are just too lazy or possess a feeling of self-entitlement that others should do for them. But I came to realize this may be the case in only a small number of cases. I came to realize that the issue of "trying" and "not doing" was actually a cultural one.

How can we be expected to do for ourselves when we are raised to look to others to take care of us (parents), to heal us (doctors), to train us (coaches) and to relax us (therapists)? Even if we want to do for ourselves, many of us just don't know how.

It is a matter of mindset. Patients must first come to accept the following five facts:

1. Health and illness are at opposite ends of a continuum;
2. Health is a process that takes time;
3. Most of the healing happens during person time, not doctors' visits;
4. The oneness for doing the daily "things" fall on the shoulders of the individual; and
5. You can change your outcomes once you change your mind.

Let's look at each of these a bit more.

THE HEALTH AND ILLNESS CONTINUUM

Optimal health and death lie at opposite ends of a wellness continuum. There are many segments between these two extremes, and illness often does not come on suddenly without several steps being crossed first. This is especially the case with regard to chronic conditions. You don't wake up with chronic headaches, for example. The head pain began for a reason and then was left to continue on until it became chronic. Often, this is the case even when one takes medication for the headache because the cause of the pain is left unchanged. Covering the pain does nothing to stop it from reoccurring again and again.

THE HEALTH PROCESS

Because health and illness are on a continuum, getting "better" is a process that takes time. Nothing is fast and permanent. There can be fast restoring of blood sugar, but the results will not be permanent unless additional actions are taken. Pain relief can be fast, but the pain will return until something more is done about the issue.

Getting healthy takes time because a process of healing is involved, which includes doing the following correctly over time:

- Sleeping
- Exercising
- Relaxing
- Taking medications and then weaning off them
- Supplementing
- Eating organic and whole foods in as close to their natural state as possible

- Stretching
- And meditating or doing deep breathing of some kind, etc.

Often, one or several things must come before other in the process. For example, pain must be diminished before range of motion can be restored.

PERSONAL HEALING TIME AND RESPONSIBILITY

The healing process occurs mostly on personal time. Sure, you can see a therapist, a dietician, an acupuncturist, a physical therapist and so on. And they can help greatly. But your time with them and the time their modality is actively working between visits are miniscule compared with the rest of the hours in your life. What this means is that the speed of the healing process is largely in your hands.

Between PT visits, you must do the physical therapies three times a day as directed. You must learn to eat healthy three times per day, even when eating out. You must learn to cook healthy meals. You must take your supplements and/or medications as directed. You must control your work/life balance and your sleep/wake cycles.

The body needs time and support to heal, and you have to supply both. If you feel like things are stalled, it may be that you stunted the process by not doing what you are supposed to do daily.

CHANGE YOUR MIND ABOUT HEALTH

As I mentioned at the start, while this sounds simple, many of us just don't know how to do it. We are trained by our medical model that it is OK to do whatever it is that got us into this illness mess, as long as we take our medication to control the numbers: the blood count, blood pressure, weight, pain scale, etc. In other words, we are taught that the doctor treats our condition, not us as a whole, and that we need not take an active role in the treatment. Is it any wonder we try hard and nothing changes?

But you can learn to stop trying and start doing for yourself in positive and effective ways. For me, the shift happened once I set in my mind what I had to do. Each morning, I have to brush my teeth. I don't try to brush my teeth, I just brush them no matter what. It is part of my daily routine. I also have needed to go to a series of physical therapy appointments. I didn't try to get to them, I just got there. I made it a point. While I needed physical therapy, I made "going to PT" a part of my daily schedule around which other things in my life were planned. The same happened with how and what I ate, when I went to sleep and woke up and when and how I exercised.

Make a list of what you know or have been asked to do for your health conditions, chronic and acute. Next to each of them write down the process involved. For example, next to "eating better" write something like "shop organic, no packaged foods, no trans fats and more vegetables." As another example, next to "exercise more" you could write "join the gym, walk at the park, get a bike buddy, join Pilates class."

In each case, you write down what needs to be done overall and then write down the specifics. Then take a look at it all and decide how best to integrate this into a weekly schedule. For me, this meant completely altering my days and weekends – in fact, my life. That was hard at first, but it became easier over time. And it is the best thing I have ever done.

Taking responsibility and placing your personal health and well-being first as priorities more important than, or at least equal to, earning a living are what it takes to control chronic conditions and prevent acute conditions from becoming chronic. If you don't see all that needs doing and then make a plan to accomplish it as needed, then you will continue to "try" to get well, overcome pain, etc., and never quite be able to "do" it all. But it all can be done by understanding the five facts and changing "trying" to "doing."

REFERENCES:

http://www.dukehealth.org/health_library/video/duke_study_acupuncture_offers_headache_relief

http://www.dukehealth.org/health_library/news/10153/

ABOUT THE AUTHOR

DR. MARK WILEY, SELF-DIRECTED WELLNESS EXPERT

*M*ark V. Wiley PhD, OMD is an internationally renowned mind-body health practitioner, author and publisher. He has spent decades traveling extensively

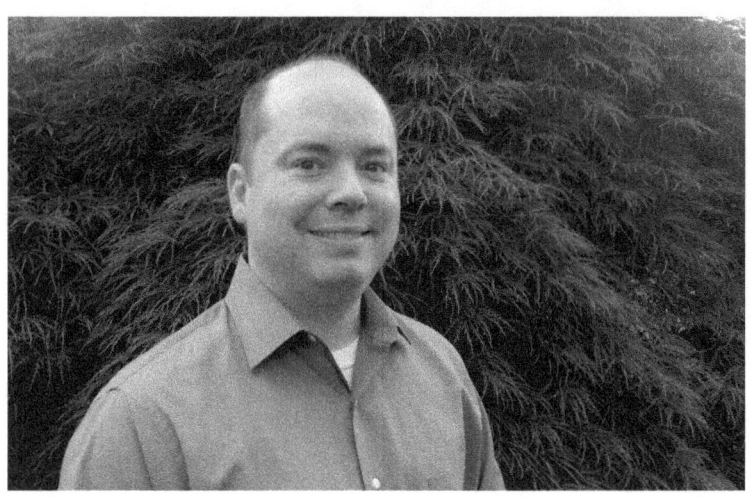

throughout the United States, Europe and Asia to research, experience, learn and master the world's alternative healing practices; from the oldest to the most modern.

Dr. Mark's interest in alternative health practices was not just a mere curiosity; he was looking for long-lasting relief from the debilitating migraines and chronic pain that plagued him from childhood. He received treatments from medical doctors, psychologists, chiropractors, physical therapists, hypnotists, acupuncturists, herbalists, bone-setters, qigong masters, yoga masters, traditional Chinese doctors, faith healers and tribal shamans. None of them, individually, were able to offer him lasting relief from his daily torment. So he took it upon himself to learn their methods, in the process earning a Master's in Health Care Management and Doctorate's in both Alternative Medicine and Oriental Medicine.

This experience and education led Dr. Mark to develop methods of uncovering root causes, relieving and then preventing – not just "treating" – physical ailments, such as migraines, back pain and arthritis, as well as conditions like hypertension, obesity, fatigue and other health concerns. His Integrated Mind-Body Approach synthesizes decades of research and personal experience, focusing on balancing the body – returning it to homeostasis – thereby providing recovery, balance and prevention of adverse health conditions. This happens because the environment that allows the condition or disease to exist is no longer present. This is the treatment that Dr. Mark used to bring his own migraines and chronic pain under control and this is the method that he promotes in his work to help others in need.

In addition to writing and publishing about health and wellness, the past decades have seen Dr. Mark interviewed for print and radio in the US, UK and Asia, lecturing at various universities, and teaching at holistic healing centers. He has written 14 books and more than 500 articles.

Today he serves on the Health Advisory Boards of several wellness centers and associations while focusing his attention on helping people achieve healthy and balanced lives through his work with Easy Health Options® and his company, Tambuli Media.

INDEX

A

Achilles tendonitis 131
acidic foods 34
acupressure 61, 128, 130
Acupressure 130
acupuncture 1, 2, 47, 59, 61,
    63, 130, 147, 181, 182, 188,
    192, 201, 202, 203, 204,
    205, 206, 208, 238
acupuncturist 2, 45, 67, 206,
    236
acute pain 2, 21, 58, 70
adductors 115, 117
adenosine triphosphate 91, 162
adrenalin 38
AIDS 106
Albany Medical Center 153,
    167
alcohol 26, 150, 165, 180, 184,
    191
alertness 27
allopathic 192
alternative medicine 1, 176, 187
Alzheimer's 138
Amazon.com 90

American Medical Association
    (AMA) 206
American Pain Foundation 24
American Society for
    Anesthesiology 205
analgesic 10, 86, 98, 100, 101,
    115, 136, 169, 191
anemic 17
Anesthesia & Analgesia 52
angelica root 12
ankles 16
Annals of the Rheumatic
    Diseases 106
antibacterial 101
antifungals 88
anti-inflammatory 3, 10, 13,
    44, 47, 62, 83, 86, 88, 97,
    98, 101, 115, 121, 125, 126,
    134, 135, 136, 138, 149,
    188, 191, 208
antioxidant 83, 88, 124, 160
antipyretic 96
antispasmodic 98, 101
antiviral properties 101

anxiety 8, 74, 102, 108, 127, 165, 166, 196, 198
arms 33, 38, 55, 57, 59, 80, 113, 114, 207, 216, 223
arnica 12, 134
aromatherapy 98, 100, 102
arthritis 1, 79, 84, 85, 87, 89, 90, 94, 95, 103, 122, 125, 129, 133, 136, 138, 171, 172, 173, 174, 175, 176, 191, 240
Arthritis Care & Research 39
Arthritis Reversed 122
Arthritis & Rheumatism 106
arthroscopic surgery 172
artificial-light exposure 28
Asia 99, 240, 241
Asian 99, 219, 220, 223
atoms 47
aura 142, 150, 151, 152, 157, 159, 161

B

back 8, 9, 11, 17, 23, 43, 46, 48, 51, 56, 59, 61, 63, 65, 71, 74, 75, 80, 81, 95, 96, 106, 107, 108, 109, 110, 111, 112, 113, 114, 115, 116, 117, 118, 119, 122, 126, 131, 135, 141, 150, 157, 168, 179, 188, 191, 192, 195, 196, 206, 207, 208, 209, 210, 211, 212, 213, 214, 216, 219, 226, 227, 240
back pain 8, 11, 43, 48, 51, 56, 59, 65, 95, 106, 107, 108, 109, 110, 114, 115, 118, 126, 188, 192, 195, 196, 208, 240
bacteria 108, 164
bending 20, 107, 118, 221
Berman, Nancy 154
beta blockers 158
Biller, José MD 151, 152
biofeedback 59, 74
bisphenol A 154
bladder 58, 88
blood 12, 13, 16, 17, 18, 20, 21, 33, 34, 35, 37, 38, 42, 46, 52, 59, 62, 65, 67, 71, 73, 80, 81, 91, 95, 96, 97, 98, 99, 100, 101, 102, 107, 108, 115, 130, 132, 133, 135, 147, 150, 151, 159, 160, 161, 166, 172, 174, 180, 181, 182, 191, 196, 206, 215, 235, 237
blood clots 99, 151
blood pressure 34, 38, 95, 237
body fluids 21, 42, 46
bodywork 2, 45, 64, 67, 79, 80, 81, 214, 215, 217, 224
bone spurs 57, 58, 131
BPA Free 155, 156
brain 23, 46, 57, 84, 94, 97, 108, 150, 151, 152, 153, 155, 157, 161
breath 40, 41, 219
breathing 34, 59, 74, 166, 236
Bristol, Terry 87
bruising 67, 98, 179

burns 83, 88
B vitamins 108, 159

C

caffeine 26, 28, 148, 165
calcium 90, 108, 158, 161
calcium channel blockers 158
camphor 12, 79, 95, 96, 98, 99
Canada 155
cancer 78, 83, 101, 103, 105, 138, 192
capsaicin 79, 82, 83, 84, 85, 95, 97, 103
capsicum 12
carbohydrates 91, 160, 164
carpal tunnel 128, 131
cartilage 57, 89, 112, 124, 137, 173
cayenne pepper 83
cell 19, 49, 88, 124, 137
cellular level 136, 137
Center for Headache and Pain Medicine 156
Centers for Disease Control and Prevention (CDC) 77
central nervous system 32, 34, 87, 123
Cerena Transcranial Magnetic Stimulator (TMS) 157
C fibers 89, 103, 124
chamomile 47
China 155, 181, 205, 214, 219
chiropractic 2, 4, 45, 46, 192, 207, 208, 225
chiropractor 2, 45, 46, 60, 62

chronic pain 1, 7, 18, 23, 24, 25, 26, 28, 31, 32, 33, 34, 36, 39, 59, 78, 81, 113, 127, 197, 199, 240, 241
cinnamon 98
circadian clock 27
circulation 17, 80, 95, 98, 115, 124, 151, 161, 180, 181, 182
Clean Energy Act of 2007 156
Clinical Orthopaedics and Related Research 49
clots 87, 99, 151
clove 98
cognitive therapies 78, 81
cold therapy 10
collagen 89, 124
College of Physicians and Surgeons at Columbia University 215
compact fluorescent bulbs (CFLs) 156
complementary exercise 42
compressing 207
connective tissue 19, 33, 48, 67, 81, 89, 124, 128, 196, 215, 216, 217
constipation 93, 127, 164, 197
Cornell University 91
cortisone 88
counterirritants 94
cramps 59, 69, 70, 95, 220
curcumin 35, 64, 83
cytokines 48, 50, 52

D

dairy 34, 148, 161, 164

dehydrated 70
deoxyribonucleic acid (DNA) 91
depression 8, 24, 25, 35, 36, 37, 40, 108, 143, 152, 165
DHA 35, 162
diabetes 8, 72, 91, 129, 133
Diamond, Seymour 151
diarrhea 102, 144, 161
diet 2, 3, 13, 36, 61, 72, 75, 81, 93, 108, 125, 135, 147, 164, 165, 166, 173, 174, 191, 224
digestion 102, 164
digestive 12, 31, 145, 164, 165, 167
discs 56, 57, 58, 60, 108
diseases 7, 100, 105, 133, 138, 164
disinfectant 96
dislocations 122
Dit Da Jow 180
diuretics 70, 165
DMSO (dimethyl sulfoxide) 86
doctor of osteopathy (DO) 224
dragon blood resin 98
Dugas, Dale Dr. 180
Duke University 201, 202, 205
Duke University Medical Center 205
dull 17, 18, 32

E

electrons 47, 157
electro-stimulation 2
elevating 35, 78
emotional disorders 32, 35
emotional freedom technique (EFT) 60
endorphins 37, 38
Energy Independence and Security Act of 2007 156
EPA 35, 162
eReader 27
essential oils 98, 99, 100
eucalyptus 94, 98
Europeans 82
Evidence-Based Complementary and Alternative Medicine 42
exercise 13, 28, 34, 36, 37, 38, 39, 42, 45, 52, 75, 78, 79, 81, 88, 115, 126, 164, 165, 166, 173, 176, 216, 238
eye movement desensitization and reprocessing (EMDR) 60

F

face 16, 166
fascia 19, 20, 21, 131, 132, 133, 135, 136, 215, 216, 217
fatigue 31, 143, 226, 240
fats 34, 35, 148, 237
Feldenkrais, Moshé 219, 220, 221, 222, 223
femur 112, 117
fever 95, 197, 198
feverfew 12
fiber 34
fibromyalgia 31, 32, 33, 34, 39, 40, 42, 43, 48, 49, 50, 51, 53, 127, 197

fingers 44, 57, 64, 67, 128, 129, 204
flat feet 133, 135
foam roller 21
folate 159
folic acid 159, 161
Food and Drug Administration (FDA) 86, 155
forehead 101
Fox, Barry 92
FOX News 156
France 155
frankincense 99
Frieden, Thomas, CDC Director 77, 78
fruits 34, 72, 148, 165
FSM therapy 48, 51

G

gait 133, 134
Gan, Tong Joo Dr. 204, 205
gastrointestinal 9, 72, 161
gating 94
gels 78, 79, 95, 100, 176, 190, 191
genes 43, 152
ginger 4, 82, 85, 86, 103, 125, 191
glucose 108
gluteal 111
gluten 164
gravity 112, 124, 214, 216, 217, 218
Green, Mark MD 125, 156
gua sha 64, 66

H

hamstrings 111, 115, 118, 119, 126
hands 3, 4, 20, 41, 55, 57, 58, 63, 69, 79, 81, 114, 118, 128, 129, 130, 212, 222, 223, 225, 236
headache 8, 95, 101, 127, 142, 144, 145, 146, 147, 148, 149, 153, 155, 157, 158, 162, 163, 164, 166, 167, 187, 197, 202, 203, 235, 238
Headache and Migraine Biology and Management 151
head posture 111
Healing Back Pain 197
health assessment 15
healthcare provider 73, 93, 109, 139, 146, 147, 149
health history 15
heart disease 7, 25, 83, 105, 106, 145, 154, 166
heat therapy 10
heel pain 133, 135, 136
herbalist 45
herbs 1, 40, 82, 180, 181, 182, 183, 184
herniated 57
high arches 133, 135
high heels 112, 133, 135
hilot 214
hinge joint 122
hip flexors 112, 113, 115
hips 33, 46, 60, 110, 111, 113, 115, 116, 117, 118, 131, 216, 223, 227

holistic 147, 174, 176, 191, 205, 206, 224, 241
homeostasis 145, 240
homeostatic 7
homocysteine 159, 160
hormones 129, 154, 165, 166
hot baths 64
house cleaning 26
hydrated 119
hydrochloric acid 102
hydrogenated oils 34
hyperextension 111
hyperlordosis 111
hypertension 91, 240
hypnotherapy 74
hypoalgesia 38
hypokalemia 72

I

ibuprofen 10, 146
Icahn School of Medicine at Mount Sinai 156
image-guided 153
immune system 123, 166
Indian Ayurvedic medicine 82
infections 32, 108, 166, 187

inflammation 1, 2, 3, 8, 10, 11, 12, 32, 34, 35, 43, 46, 47, 48, 51, 52, 62, 64, 70, 71, 73, 78, 80, 82, 83, 85, 86, 87, 88, 89, 90, 93, 94, 95, 96, 98, 103, 107, 108, 110, 122, 123, 124, 125, 127, 129, 130, 131, 132, 133, 134, 135, 137, 138, 139, 145, 146, 161, 164, 166, 172, 174, 179, 180, 187, 191, 192, 227
injury 3, 18, 19, 20, 44, 61, 67, 69, 80, 83, 105, 107, 136, 138, 139, 164, 173, 179, 180, 181, 182, 183, 198, 215, 216, 227
insomnia 25, 26, 32, 35, 74, 75
intention 40, 41
intestines 144
intranasal sphenopalatine ganglion (SPG) 153
iron 90, 108
irritable bowel syndrome (IBS) 48, 127, 197

J

joints 16, 17, 19, 20, 97, 98, 108, 111, 112, 116, 122, 127, 136, 137, 139, 172, 173, 223
Journal of Bodywork and Movement Therapies 49
Journal of Rheumatology 137

Journal of Strength and Conditioning Research 137

K

Kansas University (KU) Medical Center 154
kidney 3, 48, 72, 145, 165
kinesthetic 222
knee joint 122, 126, 127

L

lavender 98
LED lights 156
licorice 98
lidocaine 153
ligaments 58, 67, 107, 108, 122, 132, 133, 227
ligands 96
liver 3, 12, 48, 145, 160, 164, 169
low back pain (LBP) 106
Loyola University Medical Center 151
lupus 129
lymph 42, 46, 80, 130
lymphatic system 65

M

magnesium 46, 47, 71, 72, 75, 90, 91, 92, 93, 108, 161
Malaysians 82
Mandato, Kenneth MD 153, 167
martial 41

massage 4, 21, 45, 46, 59, 60, 64, 66, 80, 81, 101, 109, 115, 135, 146, 147, 181, 192, 208, 214, 217, 218, 222
Mauskop, Alexander 92
medical iv, 1, 4, 18, 23, 31, 41, 42, 44, 61, 69, 82, 87, 107, 121, 122, 139, 141, 147, 158, 174, 176, 179, 187, 188, 192, 198, 201, 202, 204, 224, 237, 240
meditation 36, 59, 60, 74, 146, 191, 219, 221
meditative 40, 42, 220
melatonin 27, 28
menopause 129
menses 85
menthol 79, 94, 95, 96, 98, 100, 101
meridians 51, 61, 175, 203
microcurrent technology 48
migraine 9, 32, 35, 91, 92, 142, 143, 146, 147, 149, 150, 151, 152, 153, 154, 156, 157, 158, 159, 160, 161, 162, 167, 168, 169, 188, 197, 202
migraine spray 167
mindful exercise 42
mint 95, 96, 182
misaligned 45, 60
molecular level 43
movement 20, 21, 33, 41, 42, 46, 56, 60, 65, 67, 113, 122, 126, 135, 137, 138, 165, 217, 219, 220, 221, 222, 223
MRI 190

muscle 1, 2, 3, 12, 13, 17, 19, 39, 46, 47, 48, 60, 61, 63, 64, 65, 66, 69, 70, 71, 72, 73, 74, 75, 80, 81, 89, 98, 99, 100, 101, 110, 111, 112, 113, 114, 115, 125, 130, 146, 148, 209, 210, 211, 214, 220, 221, 223, 224, 225, 226, 227, 228
muscle contraction 130, 146
muscle strain 101
musculoskeletal 1, 85, 103, 127, 188, 196, 197
myofascial 48, 66
myofascial release 66
myrrh 99

N

naproxen 10
National Headache Foundation 151
Native Americans 82
natural 1, 2, 4, 8, 10, 12, 18, 21, 23, 24, 33, 35, 38, 40, 43, 44, 45, 52, 53, 60, 72, 77, 81, 82, 83, 96, 98, 101, 108, 110, 122, 123, 125, 131, 134, 135, 138, 154, 162, 174, 175, 187, 188, 191, 192, 193, 204, 216, 221, 235
naturopathic medicine 100
nausea 85, 95, 142, 150, 151, 205

neck 8, 10, 11, 17, 43, 46, 55, 56, 57, 58, 59, 60, 61, 62, 63, 74, 85, 101, 103, 166, 179, 206, 207, 216, 227
neck pain 10, 43, 55, 56, 57, 58, 59, 60, 61, 62, 63, 85, 103, 206
nerve pain 43, 44, 45, 46, 47, 52, 96
nerves 17, 33, 43, 44, 45, 46, 56, 57, 58, 60, 75, 79, 80, 84, 96, 97, 98, 107, 168, 196, 215
neuro-linguistic programming (NLP) 60
neuropathic pain 45, 46, 51, 52
neurotransmitter NMDA 46
New York Headache Center 162
nightshades 3
nitrates 148, 150, 164
Norwegian University of Science and Technology at St. Olav University Hospital 37
NSAIDs (nonsteroidal anti-inflammatory drugs) 44, 62, 208
numbness 44, 46, 48, 58, 128, 129, 196
nutritionist 45

O

obesity 8, 129, 240
occiput 101
ointments 78, 124, 136

opioids 24, 78, 205
Oregon Health Sciences University 87
organ 19, 61, 71, 87, 162, 217
organic 3, 96, 173, 235, 237
orthotic 135
osteoarthritis (OA) 84, 85
over-the-counter (OTC) 9
oxygen 21, 33, 38, 59, 65, 70, 73, 91, 101, 108, 115, 160, 166, 196
oxygen deprivation 59, 166

P

painkillers 77, 78, 81, 145, 188, 204
pain patches 10, 69
pain syndrome 11, 12, 13, 31
palpating 62
pancreatitis 72
paraspinal muscles 45
patient consultation 15
pelvis 111, 116, 135, 227
penicillin 88
peppermint 95, 96, 98, 99, 100, 101, 102
peripheral nervous system 44
phosphorous 90
physical examination 15, 35, 49
physical therapist 2, 222, 236
physical therapy 2, 66, 67, 78, 173, 190, 208, 228, 237
Pilates 238
pillows 63
PLOS ONE 25
podiatrist 135, 136

posture 41, 55, 57, 59, 60, 63, 75, 101, 110, 111, 112, 113, 114, 135, 207, 214, 215, 218, 220
potassium 72, 73, 75, 90, 108
pregnancy 129
Proceedings of the National Academy of Sciences of the United States of America 27
proprioceptive neuromuscular facilitation (PNF) 225
prostaglandin 95
psychosomatic 126, 196, 197, 218

Q

qi (energy) 17, 41
qigong 33, 40, 41, 42, 43, 59, 74, 191, 219, 240
quadratus lumborum (QL) 118
quadriceps 115, 118, 126
quantum touch 47

R

randomized controlled trials (RCT) 42
range of motion 4, 11, 19, 33, 48, 55, 56, 62, 79, 81, 110, 112, 113, 115, 130, 136, 137, 138, 172, 191, 206, 216, 217, 221, 222, 223, 224, 225, 226, 227, 228, 236
rebound 145, 227
rebound pain 145, 227

recommended daily allowance (RDA) 23
recovery 20, 25, 50, 205, 233, 240
red flower oil 98
red wine 148
relaxation 41, 46, 81, 146, 192
religious 41
REM sleep 27
repetitive inactivity 19
Resnicj, Lawrence MD 91
rest 57, 90, 111, 134, 135, 172, 191, 236
resting 13, 17, 101, 115
rheumatism 85, 95, 99, 103
rheumatoid arthritis (RA) 84, 85
ribonucleic acid (RNA) 91
Rolf, Ida Dr. 215, 216, 217

S

salicylates 95, 96
Sarno, John MD 195, 197
scapular muscles 59
scar tissue 33, 48, 81
Schechter, David MD 198, 199
sciatica 18, 43, 46, 95
sciatic nerve 116, 117
s-curve 110
sedative 96
sedentary 135, 172, 173
Sedona Method 60
self-acupressure 130
shingles 48, 51
shoes 112, 133, 135, 221

shoulders 17, 20, 33, 46, 55, 56, 57, 58, 59, 61, 62, 64, 101, 111, 165, 166, 206, 207, 208, 211, 214, 216, 227, 234
sinus 164, 203
skeletal system 175
skeletal trauma 108
skin 19, 44, 49, 51, 65, 66, 67, 71, 87, 88, 89, 94, 95, 97, 98, 100, 101, 102, 124, 181
sleep 2, 21, 23, 24, 25, 26, 27, 28, 29, 32, 34, 36, 42, 55, 62, 75, 102, 112, 132, 142, 143, 144, 147, 148, 150, 164, 165, 166, 167, 191, 236, 237
sleep deprivation 25, 167
sleeping posture 59, 60, 63
Society of Interventional Radiology 153, 167
sodas 70
sodium 108
Spain 34
spasms 1, 11, 45, 46, 47, 64, 66, 69, 70, 71, 73, 74, 75, 89, 112, 125, 221, 223
spices 3, 82, 86, 125, 161, 191
spinal health 110, 225
spine 2, 4, 17, 45, 46, 49, 60, 65, 73, 75, 101, 108, 111
spirit 24, 32
sports 55, 58, 63, 66, 110, 122, 179, 228
sprains 87, 88, 98, 99, 122, 124, 136
spurs 57, 58, 122, 131
squatting 20

stabbing pain 17
Star, Michael MD 151, 152
stasis 16, 17
State University of New York Empire State College 153
steroid injections 121
stiffness 16, 61, 63, 64, 78, 88, 93, 94, 97, 138, 191, 196, 206, 207, 216, 221, 227
stimuli 16
St. John's wort 35
stomach 9, 12, 59, 85, 100, 102, 112, 114, 144, 150
stress 8, 25, 32, 35, 40, 55, 59, 61, 62, 63, 73, 74, 75, 83, 101, 102, 123, 127, 132, 133, 134, 135, 142, 147, 148, 150, 164, 165, 166, 167, 196, 198, 207, 214, 216, 217, 218
stretching 4, 13, 21, 33, 63, 73, 115, 146, 208, 225
stroke 87, 150, 151, 152, 154, 160
subluxation 63
substance P 84, 85, 97
sugar 3, 34, 148, 150, 164, 191, 235
sulfur 89, 124
sunlight 70
surgery 8, 121, 125, 128, 130, 131, 172, 191, 192, 205
swayback 110, 111, 112, 113, 114
sweating 97, 165, 203
symptomatic relief 2, 8, 12, 50, 100, 131
symptoms 2, 7, 8, 9, 11, 12, 13, 15, 18, 31, 32, 33, 40, 42, 43, 46, 57, 87, 89, 92, 94, 95, 97, 101, 115, 121, 123, 127, 131, 134, 138, 142, 145, 146, 147, 155, 157, 158, 163, 168, 171, 172, 173, 175, 176, 190, 195, 196, 197, 198, 199, 203

T

tai chi 33, 59, 219
temporal mandibular joint dysfunction (TMJD) 127, 197
tension headache 127, 197
tension myositis syndrome (TMS) 60
tensor fasciae latae (TFL) 116
TENS units 47, 51, 63
Thai yoga massage 214
The Global Burden of Disease Study 105
The Journal of Physiology 46
The Lancet 105
The MindBody Workbook 199
The National Institutes of Health 25
thermogenic 86, 191
thighs 111
tightness 13, 62, 64, 67, 100, 101, 110, 130, 146, 190, 206, 207, 208, 227
tingling 44, 46, 58, 128, 129, 196
tinnitus 127, 197

toes 20, 44, 131
topical analgesics 88
topical creams 78, 81, 96
topical pain 79, 88, 124, 191
toxins 21, 23, 33, 71, 73, 148, 164
traction devices 63
traditional Chinese medicine (TCM) 82, 89, 98, 130, 146, 179
trans fats 34, 237
trauma 3, 32, 33, 44, 49, 55, 58, 88, 108, 123, 129, 179, 180, 182, 183
trigger points 1, 3, 10, 11, 13, 42, 46, 48, 66, 80, 110, 112, 146, 208, 223
triptans 158
Tui Na 181, 225
turmeric 4, 12, 82, 83, 86, 125, 134, 191
turpentine 98

U

ultrasound 47
University of Connecticut 137
University of New South Wales and Neuroscience Research Australia 38

V

valerian 64
vasoconstriction 35, 91, 97
vasodilation 96
vegetables 34, 72, 85, 125, 148, 160, 161, 165, 237

Vermeer, Lydia 154, 155
vertebrae 45, 56, 57, 62
viruses 32, 108
visual analog scale (VAS) 50
visualizations 74
vitamin D3 47

W

walking 26, 33, 34, 73, 118, 132, 190, 216
water 16, 34, 70, 71, 75, 119, 155, 156, 165
water aerobics 34
water bottles 155
weight 36, 60, 81, 111, 114, 122, 127, 133, 135, 237
wellbeing 42, 55, 114
What Your Doctor May Not Tell You About Migraines 92
wheat 3, 72, 164
whiplash 61
whole grains 34, 72, 162, 165
wintergreen 94, 95, 96, 98
Wong Lop Kong Medicated Oil 79, 99
World Health Organization (WHO) 188
wrists 16, 102

Y

yoga 33, 34, 59, 60, 73, 74, 81, 115, 191, 214, 219, 240

Z

zinc 90, 108

ARTHRITIS REVERSED
2ND EDITION

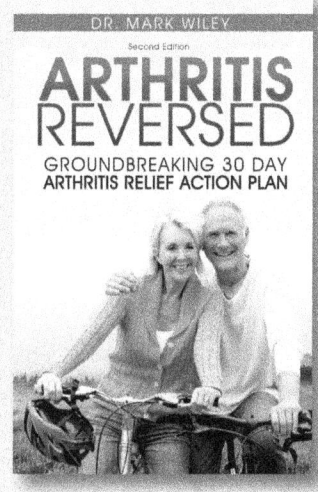

Dr. Mark Wiley has spent decades researching and mastering natural wellness practices around the world. He's taken those techniques and pioneered a powerful, integrated mind/body approach to arthritis relief and prevention. Simply put, mainstream medicine fails to eradicate our everyday pains, illnesses and diseases. It fails because it is *passive* and *reactionary* and thus it is unable to prevent you from experiencing chronic health conditions. The important thing is to see and know that the solution to your daily suffering is grounded in a five-part process called, the ***Arthritis Relief Action Plan:***

Part 1: Educate yourself about the real causes and solutions of arthritis
Part 2: Reduce the current level of symptoms you are experiencing
Part 3: Halt or significantly reduce the worsening of your condition
Part 4: Prevent the symptoms from flaring to improve your quality of life
Part 5: Regenerate healthy tissue to reverse the damage done

In the pages of ***Arthritis Reversed***, Dr. Wiley shows you how to determine the underlying—and sometimes hidden—causes of your arthritic symptoms. These are actually obvious root causes and contributors that are only "hidden" because you have not (yet) been taught to look for and identify them. Dr. Wiley shows you how to do this and then how to use that knowledge to reduce your pain and halt or slow the progression of the condition, typically within 30 to 90 days.

> "*Arthritis Reversed* is a road map to recovery from arthritic pain and will help you get your life back." —*Dr. Robert del Medico*
>
> "Do not let Arthritis rule your life! Get this book and see what it can do for you. It has helped my patients gain more control over their lives." —*Dr. Dale Dugas*
>
> "Dr. Wiley explains the biggest mistakes made in treating arthritis, and the inflammatory response. I highly recommend this book to anyone suffering from any form of arthritis." —*Dr. Robert Chu*

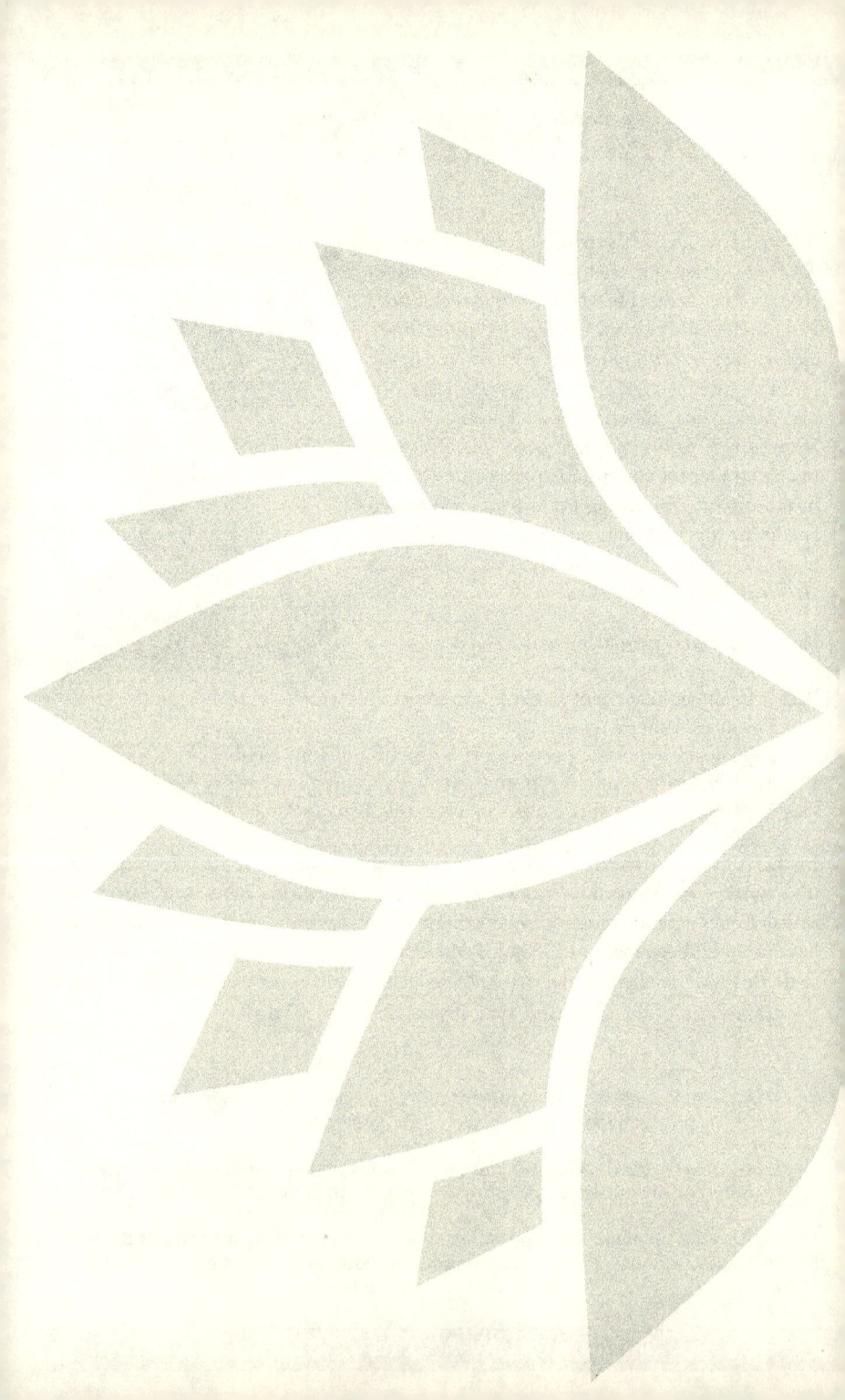

HEADACHES RELIEVED
30-Days to Lasting Relief from Headaches & Migraines

After suffering debilitating migraines and headaches every day for 30 years Dr. Mark Wiley woke up and decided he'd had enough. After a lifetime of suffering, followed by decades of advanced study and intensive travel to meet with traditional healers and medical experts the world over, Dr. Wiley was able to overcome his chronic headaches and migraines.

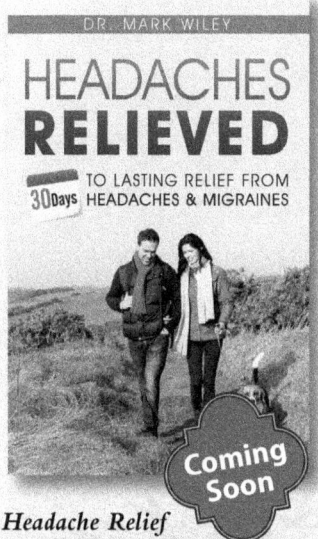

You, too, can relieve your headaches once and for all. In the pages of *Headaches Relieved*, Dr. Wiley presents the program to help you get rid of the crushing, throbbing pain forever. Whether your headaches are cluster or migraine, stress-induced or vascular, allergic or rebound, you will find relief in this simple program that allows you to see and know that the solution to your daily suffering is grounded in a five-part process Dr. Wiley calls, the *Headache Relief Action Plan*:

Part 1: Educate yourself about the real causes and solutions for headaches and migraines
Part 2: Reduce the current level of painful symptoms you are experiencing
Part 3: Halt or significantly reduce the frequency and duration of your headaches
Part 4: Prevent the headaches from triggering to improve your quality of life
Part 5: Repair the body to reduce the internal environment that allows for headaches

In the pages of *Headaches Relieved*, Dr. Wiley shows you how to determine the underlying — and sometimes hidden — causes of your headaches and migraines. These are actually obvious root causes and contributors that are only "hidden" because you have not (yet) been taught to look for and identify them. Dr. Wiley shows you how to do this and then how to use that knowledge to halt or slow the frequency and reduce the intensity and duration of your headaches, typically within 30 days. Empower yourself to end your pain today!

> "Dr. Wiley's compelling story and self-directed program will give any headache sufferer the belief: If he can do it, so can I! This book is essential."
> —*Dr. Brett Cardonick*

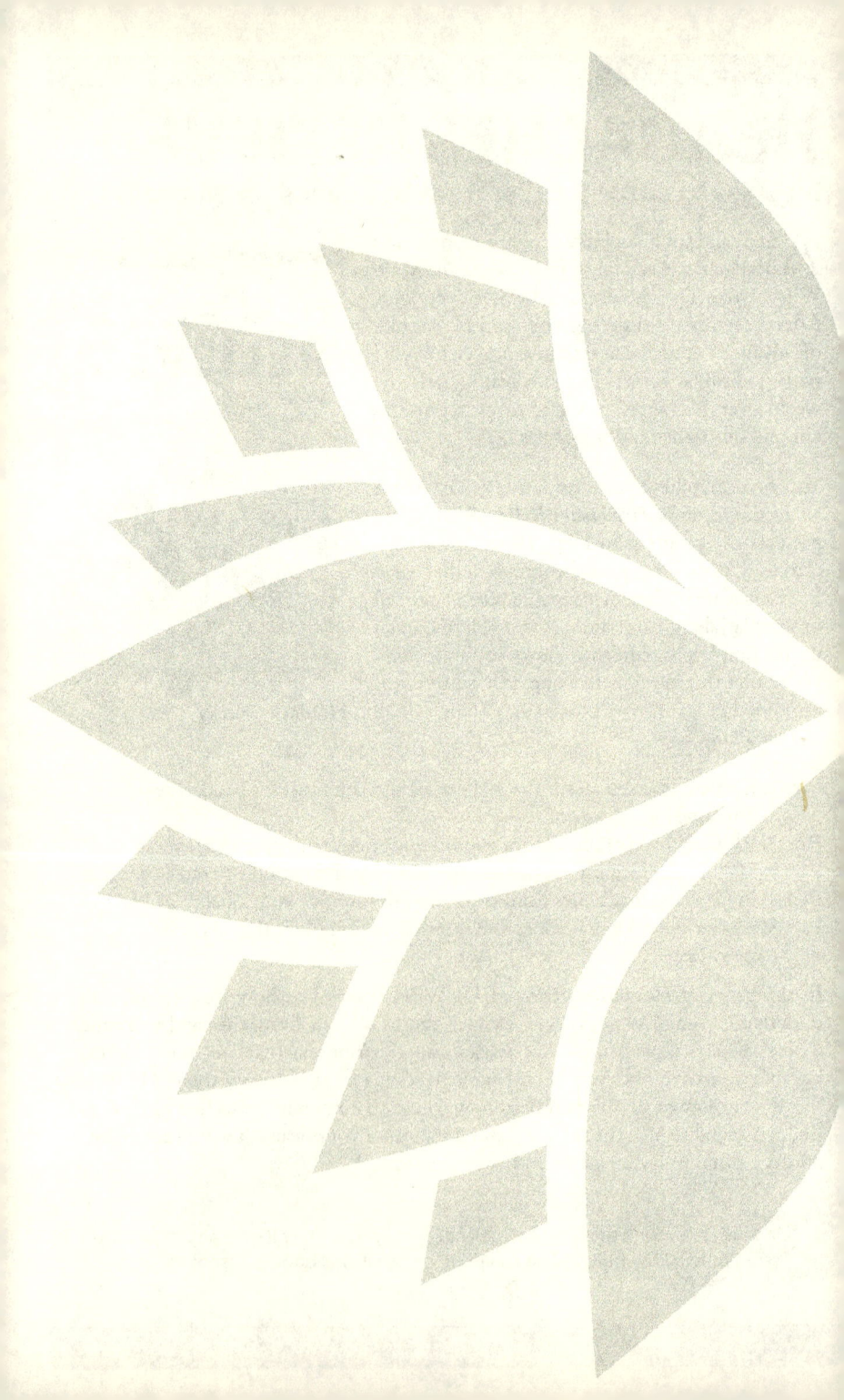

www.ingramcontent.com/pod-product-compliance
Lightning Source LLC
Chambersburg PA
CBHW031145020426
42333CB00013B/515